Alcohol and Sport

Robert D. Stainback, PhD

Birmingham Department of Veterans Affairs
Medical Center

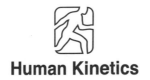

Human Kinetics

Library of Congress Cataloging-in-Publication Data

Stainback, Robert D., 1954-
    Alcohol and sport / Robert D. Stainback.
       p.   cm.
    Includes bibliographical references (p.) and index.
    ISBN 0-87322-531-7
    1. Athletes--Alcohol use.   I. Title.
    RC1245.S73   1997   96-48332
    616.86'1'0088796--dc21   CIP

ISBN: 0-87322-531-7

Photo Credits: Chapter 1, © Unicorn/Jim Shipee; Chapter 2, © Unicorn/Joseph Sohm; Chapter 3, © Unicorn/Jim Shipee; Chapter 4, © Mary Langenfeld; Chapter 5, © Terry Wild Studio; Chapter 6, © Unicorn/Aneal Vohra; Chapter 7, © Terry Wild Studio; Chapter 8, © Unicorn/Aneal Vohra

Acquisitions Editor: Richard D. Frey, PhD; **Developmental Editor**: Marni Basic; **Assistant Editors**: John Wentworth and Alesha G. Thompson; **Editorial Assistant**: Amy Carnes; **Copyeditor**: Denelle Eknes; **Proofreader**: Sue Fetters; **Indexer**: Mary Prottsman; **Graphic Designer**: Robert Reuther; **Graphic Artist**: Sandra Meier; **Photo Editor**: Boyd LaFoon; **Cover Designer**: Keith Blomberg; **Photographer** (cover): Michael Moffett; **Illustrator**: Sara Wolfsmith; **Composition**: Braun-Brumfield; **Printer**: Braun-Brumfield

Printed in the United States of America   10   9   8   7   6   5   4   3   2   1

Human Kinetics
Web site: http://www.humankinetics.com/

United States: Human Kinetics, P.O. Box 5076, Champaign, IL 61825-5076
1-800-747-4457
e-mail: humank@hkusa.com

Canada: Human Kinetics, Box 24040, Windsor, ON N8Y 4Y9
1-800-465-7301 (in Canada only)
e-mail: humank@hkcanada.com

Europe: Human Kinetics, P.O. Box IW14, Leeds LS16 6TR, United Kingdom
(44) 1132 781708
e-mail: humank@hkeurope.com

Australia: Human Kinetics, 57A Price Avenue, Lower Mitcham, South Australia 5062
(08) 277 1555
e-mail: humank@hkaustralia.com

New Zealand: Human Kinetics, P.O. Box 105-231, Auckland 1
(09) 523 3462
e-mail: humank@hknewz.com

To my wife, Judy,
an eternal source of love and joy.

CONTENTS

4

Alcohol Abuse and Dependence Among Athletes and Sport Professionals   71

5

Sport-Related Alcohol Abuse and Dependence Prevention   99

Contents

PREFACE

Alcohol use is common in the United States and many other nations. In many societies, heavy drinking is condoned, either implicitly through a pervasive lack of attention to the detrimental effects of alcohol abuse or explicitly through advertising. While one might think that athletes and others involved in sport and physical activity would be less susceptible to the negative effects of alcohol and other drugs, this is often not the case. In fact, along with the general association of alcohol with leisure—many people tend to link drinking alcohol with living the good life—athletes, sports fans, and other participants in physical activity can have additional motivations for drinking. Although it's true that active people are more likely than the sedentary to know what is good and bad for their bodies, it's also true that the sport arena and physical activity have a long-standing association with alcohol. You see this association most extremely in spectators of sport, who often drink while they watch, sometimes viewing an athletic event as an opportunity for drinking more than they would otherwise. But the participants themselves are also likely to use alcohol, often for sport-related reasons, though generally after the event has ended. Among many other possible motivations, sport or physical activity participants might drink to celebrate a victory, relax and wind down, or console themselves after a loss or poor performance.

In this book I'll focus on the task of the professional (e.g., sport psychologists, athletic trainers, sport physical therapists, sport-related physicians, and sport management and administrative specialists) involved in minimizing the detrimental effects of alcohol on athletes and, indirectly, all individuals who appreciate sport and who are influenced by the behavior of athletes and others involved in sport. I assume that readers will have an interest in increasing their knowledge and ability to identify athletes with alcohol-related problems, assist them in changing their drinking habits, and, when necessary, help them to obtain professional treatment. A secondary purpose of the book is to increase the awareness of sport professionals regarding alcohol use and abuse in the sport community, including within their own ranks, and among spectators of sport events.

The book contains eight chapters. In chapter 1, I offer an overview of alcohol and addiction, including sections on alcohol use, abuse, and dependence and their epidemiology and economic costs. This chapter also covers diagnosis and associated medical and psychiatric morbidity of alcohol abuse and dependence. Sections on etiological theories and risk factors for alcohol dependence conclude the chapter.

In chapter 2, I review the history of the relation between alcohol and sport in the United States and the alcohol use patterns of the general population, athletes, sport professionals, and sport spectators. Chapter 3 describes the biomedical and behavioral effects of alcohol and their influence on human functioning and sport performance. In chapter 4, I discuss the incidence of and risk factors for alcohol abuse and dependence among athletes and sport professionals. I present several case examples of alcohol-related problems among members of these populations.

In chapter 5, methods of preventing alcohol abuse and dependence are examined. I offer specific recommendations for who in the sport community should participate in prevention efforts and what actions they should take. Chapter 6 addresses methods to help the problem drinker change. This chapter advises the professional who does not have specialized training in addiction treatment but would like information on how problem drinkers make positive changes in their drinking behavior and ways that concerned professionals may help.

In chapter 7, I describe characteristics of many alcohol treatment approaches, general conclusions of treatment outcome studies, and implications for treatment for athletes who abuse or depend on alcohol. Finally, in chapter 8, I review major points of previous chapters, present conclusions, and suggest some considerations for the future.

Two appendixes are included to provide an overview of alcohol use in society (Appendix A) and a resource guide for treatment and prevention of alcohol problems (Appendix B). Questions for discussion are also included to stimulate additional exploration of the topics covered in the book.

The problem of alcohol abuse among athletes and others involved in sport and physical activity is one that can be understood and overcome only through the patient diligence of professionals working with affected individuals. It is my hope that the information in this book will move you toward understanding the complex motivations for alcohol use in the sport world and assisting those who need help in overcoming alcohol-related problems.

ACKNOWLEDGMENTS

Writing a book always requires support and cooperation from countless people, and this project is no exception. I would like to recognize some of the people who helped make this book possible. I want to thank Dr. Shane Murphy for recommending to Human Kinetics that I write a book on alcohol and sport. My thanks also go to colleagues at the Birmingham Department of Veterans Affairs Medical Center who provided professional and administrative coverage during my absences to work on the manuscript, especially to Drs. Jesse Milby, Laura Whitworth, and Gloria Roque, and to Willie Fields, Ken Beard, and Sally Bakane. The Human Kinetics staff who guided me through the manuscript preparation process deserves thanks as well, particularly Marni Basic, Amy Carnes, John Wentworth, and Dr. Rick Frey. Many thanks to the external reviewers whose feedback improved the manuscript and to Gloria Brown for typing the manuscript draft. I also am grateful to my clients for the privilege of working with them in their endeavors to lead happy, productive lives. It is through that work that I acquired the knowledge and experience to compile this book. Finally, I want my family to know how much I appreciate their support during the long process of writing this book. Thank you Mom, Dad, Frank, Dave, Laura, and Nancy for your continuing love and interest in my career. Thank you Paul and Tami for your patience and understanding when I was devoting time to writing. Finally, thank you Judy for being such a sharing and caring partner, never failing to encourage me when I needed it. Thanks for keeping the faith.

1 INTRODUCTION TO ALCOHOL AND ADDICTION

Substances which act on the brain mock at all obstacles which oppose their extension. Their attraction grows slowly, silently, but surely.

—L. Lewin

This chapter provides the reader with a background regarding alcohol and addiction to its use. After defining terms commonly found in the alcohol literature, we will explore the epidemiology of alcohol use, abuse, and dependence and related economic costs. The next section describes diagnostic classification systems for alcohol abuse and dependence, followed by a review of medical and psychiatric morbidity and mortality associated with alcohol abuse and dependence. The chapter discusses various theories of etiology for alcohol dependence and concludes with a section on risk factors for alcohol dependence.

In many respects, this chapter is a primer providing the reader with the necessary information about alcohol use, abuse, and dependence to be able to appreciate and apply the following chapters to resolving alcohol-related issues in the sport context. Without the information in chapter 1, the reader would lack the context from which to evaluate alcohol use, abuse, and dependence among athletes and sport professionals.

DEFINING TERMS

Descriptions of problems related to alcohol use vary depending on which literature you read. For purposes of this book, *alcohol abuse* and *alcohol dependence* (also referred to as *alcoholism*) are disorders in which significant impairments in human functioning directly relate to a maladaptive pattern of alcohol use. Alcohol dependence is characterized by more pronounced impairments in functioning than alcohol abuse and may include evidence of physiological dependence (see the section on diagnosis in this chapter for more details). These terms are the diagnostic nomenclature in the American Psychiatric Association's *Diagnostic and Statistical Manual of Mental Disorders* (1994), now in its fourth edition (*DSM-IV*). Related terms such as substance or chemical abuse or dependence are more general and refer to abuse of or dependence on any addictive substance (e.g., alcohol, cocaine, nicotine).

The terms *problem drinking* and *problem drinker*, commonly used in behavioral psychology, describe related concepts but refer to any drinking pattern that causes problems for the drinker, regardless of whether they meet *DSM-IV* diagnostic criteria. This terminology therefore refers to a broader scope of problems related to alcohol use. *Alcohol use*, or *social drinking*, as opposed to the previous terms, refers to alcohol consumption patterns that are not associated with recurring medical, psychological, or social problems.

ALCOHOL USE, ABUSE, AND DEPENDENCE

Alcohol has a long history in civilization. Though the inception of its use is debated, alcohol as a beverage may have appeared as early as 8,000 B.C., and its use continues to be popular in a substantial part of the world today.

Indeed, alcohol is the most used psychoactive drug in many cultures. It is produced in various forms, including beers, wines, liqueurs, and distilled spirits. Each of these beverages contains increasing amounts of pure alcohol. Concentrations of alcohol are approximately 4.2 percent by volume in beers, 12 to 20 percent in wines, 22 to 50 percent in liqueurs, and 40 to 50 percent (80 to 100 proof) in distilled spirits. A standard "drink" typically contains .5 oz of pure alcohol, which corresponds approximately to 12 oz of beer, 2.5 to 4.2 oz of wine, or 1 to 1.3 oz of distilled spirits. In 1993, the apparent annual per capita alcohol consumption in the United States was 2.25 gallons of pure alcohol for those aged 14 years or older (Williams, Stinson, Stewart & Dufour, 1995). (For a point of reference, this translates to approximately 571 12-oz cans of beer annually or 11 cans per week.) Keep in mind that this figure represents an average and does not reflect alcohol consumption of individual drinkers. In reality, the majority of alcohol is consumed by a minority of the population. Five percent of U.S. adult (18 and older) drinkers consumes approximately 50 percent of the alcohol, and 25 percent of U.S. adult drinkers consumes between 87 and 89 percent of the alcohol in the United States. Younger (18–29 years old) male drinkers are largely overrepresented in the highest volume drinking categories (Greenfield, 1995). For the interested reader, appendix A (page 175) contains a brief history of alcohol use in society and an overview of contemporary alcohol use in the United States and selected other countries. This information may be helpful to the reader for appreciating the topics presented in this and other chapters.

Sociocultural variables determine initiation of alcohol use. Typically, parental drinking attitudes and habits determine if and when an individual will begin to drink. As one progresses into adolescence, peer group attitudes and behaviors about alcohol become influential in determining one's drinking habits. For most people, alcohol use does not pose a significant health threat. However, it was estimated that 15.3 million adults in the United States in 1988 (approximately 9 percent of the population over age 18) met diagnostic criteria for alcohol abuse or dependence (Grant, Harford, et al., 1991).

EPIDEMIOLOGY OF ALCOHOL USE, ABUSE, AND DEPENDENCE

Recent epidemiological data indicate per capita alcohol consumption has declined steadily in the United States from 1981 to 1993 (see figure 1.1). Decreased consumption of distilled spirits accounted for most of this decline. Possible reasons for the decline in alcohol consumption include increased public awareness of risks involved in alcohol use, growing emphasis

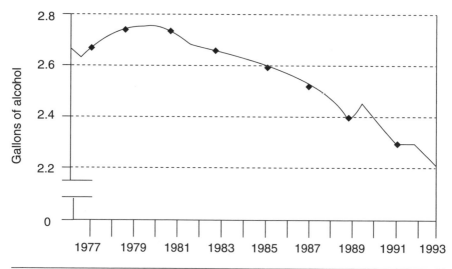

Figure 1.1 Total per capita alcohol consumption, United States, 1977–1993.

From *Apparent Per Capita Alcohol Consumption: National, State, and Regional Trends, 1977–1993* (p. 4) by G.D. Williams, F.S. Stinson, S.L. Stewart, and M.C. Dufour, 1995, Bethesda, Maryland: National Institute on Alcohol Abuse and Alcoholism.

on health and fitness, a change in the demographics, with the proportion of the population over age 60 increasing (alcohol consumption in this age group is low), and a conservative cultural climate, which is often associated with reduced tolerance for heavy drinking (U.S. Department of Health and Human Services [USDHHS], 1990). Other industrialized nations have reported similar declines in alcohol consumption. Despite these declines in use, however, alcohol remains a substantial drug of abuse in the United States and in most of the industrialized world. Furthermore, per capita drinking levels have remained elevated since relatively rapid increases occurred in the 1960s.

In reviewing recent studies on patterns of alcohol consumption, the *Seventh Special Report to the U.S. Congress on Alcohol and Health* (USDHHS, 1990) concluded that consumption patterns in the United States have remained stable from the mid-1960s through the early 1980s. One exception noted, however, was an increase in heavy drinking among young people ages 21 to 34. This trend was particularly apparent among young women who were drinkers. In general, men were more likely to drink and to be heavier drinkers than women.

A more recent study comparing alcohol consumption patterns in the United States in 1983 and 1988 (Williams & De-Bakey, 1992) corroborated the earlier finding that men were more likely to drink and to drink heavily than women. However, the study also found during this six-year period that widespread increases in abstention occurred for both men and women. Furthermore, significant decreases were found in heavier drinking across a wide range of sociodemographic variables. This recent finding suggests that heavier drinking may have peaked in the early 1980s and is now decreasing.

Longitudinal epidemiological data have indicated that the incidence of problems related to alcohol use remained stable from 1967 to 1984; however, small increases in prevalence of dependence symptoms were noted for both men and women (Hilton & Clark, 1987). A recent survey (Hilton, 1991a, 1991b) of current drinkers regarding social and other consequences of alcohol use during the past year suggested that alcohol-related problems were diverse and occurred with various levels of severity. Hilton's survey results suggested that alcohol-related problems were not confined to a small number of alcohol abusers or dependents, but occurred in many drinkers who would not necessarily meet diagnostic criteria for an alcohol use disorder (Hilton, 1991a).

ALCOHOL USE, ABUSE, AND DEPENDENCE IN SUBPOPULATIONS

A composite, modal description of heavy drinkers and those experiencing drinking-related problems (both dependence symptoms and drinking-related social and personal consequences) is male, between the ages of 18 and 29, and single (USDHHS, 1990). Drinking-related problems in men are variable over time with a high degree of remission as age increases to midlife and beyond (Fillmore, 1987), which is consistent with general decreases in consumption. It has been reliably found over time and across cultures that men drink more than women and experience more alcohol-related negative consequences (Wilsnack & Wilsnack, 1991).

Women

Although there has been recent concern that women's drinking is increasing and the gap between men's and women's drinking is narrowing, evidence in the last 20 years has suggested little overall change in women's alcohol consumption levels and related consequences. For women who drink, the most consistent predictors of onset of problem drinking appear to be youth, cohabitation, and lifetime use of drugs other than alcohol. Persistent or chronic problem drinking was associated with sexual dysfunction, part-time employment, never marrying, or experiencing recent depression (Wilsnack, Klassen, Schur, & Wilsnack, 1991). Another study found childhood sexual abuse predictive of problem drinking in women (Wilsnack, 1991).

High School Students

Comparing recent annual surveys of high school seniors indicates a decline in current alcohol use (use in the past 30 days) in this population during the 1980s and early 1990s (Johnston, O'Malley, & Bachman, 1995). Alcohol use remains at a disturbing rate, however. Eighty-seven percent of seniors in 1993 reported having tried alcohol; 51 percent were categorized as current drinkers, and 28 percent were occasional heavy drinkers (took five or more drinks at a sitting during the past two weeks) (Johnston, O'Malley, & Bachman, 1994). In the transition from adolescence to young adulthood there is little continuity in drinking patterns, and as age 30 approaches drinking levels tend to decline (Temple & Fillmore, 1985–1986). However, this level of alcohol consumption during adolescence is particularly disturbing because of recent supportive evidence for the gateway theory, which suggests that age of onset of alcohol use and frequency of use are strong predictors of progression to use of marijuana, other illicit drugs, and medically prescribed psychoactive drugs (Kandel, Yamaguchi, & Chen, 1992). This theory implies that those adolescents starting alcohol use early are at greater risk to use other drugs than are their abstinent peers.

Elderly

In general, alcohol consumption levels of persons 60 and older are lower and alcohol abuse less prevalent than in younger age groups. It is uncertain whether this lower level of alcohol consumption is from factors related to aging or to cohort effects (i.e., influences on drinking related to cultural or historical factors in each generation). Longitudinal studies (e.g., Stall, 1986) indicate that when changes in consumption do occur in older adults, they are more often decreases than increases. Therefore, there are more abstainers and fewer heavy drinkers among older adults. Frequency of drinking-related problems decreases in older adults; however, late-onset heavy drinking may occur in response to stressful life events, such as declining health, financial status changes, or retirement (Atkinson, 1988). This late-onset heavy drinking is usually a milder form of alcohol problem than early-onset alcohol abuse or dependence and is less likely to relate to a family history of alcohol dependence or of psychological disorders. It also may occur with more frequency than originally thought (Atkinson, Tolson, & Turner, 1990).

Ethnic Minorities

The four major racial and ethnic minority groups in the United States (African Americans, Hispanics, Asian Americans, and American Indian and Alaska Native tribes) may demonstrate collective patterns of alcohol use and alcohol-related problems that are distinct from the population at large. However, as described in appendix A, because of diversity in alcohol use within ethnic groups and difficulties in consistently conceptualizing ethnicity in studies, generalizations regarding alcohol use among ethnic groups must be made judiciously. With these caveats in mind, the following paragraphs address alcohol use in the four major racial and ethnic minorities in the United States.

African Americans. Recent surveys (cited in USDHHS, 1993) have indicated that African American and white males had similar drinking patterns, though African American males reported higher abstention rates. African American males also reported a higher incidence of alcohol-related problems during the prior year than white males reported, even though rates of heavy drinking among African Americans were lower. These results suggest that African American males are more vulnerable to alcohol-related problems than white males at similar or lower consumption levels. Herd (1989) speculated that this apparent higher vulnerability to alcohol-related problems among African American males may be from later onset of heavier and more sustained drinking, whereas in white males heavy drinking is more likely to be short term and associated with youth. Herd (1987) also suggested that the higher vulnerability of African American males to alcohol-related problems may be associated with social and economic difficulties, such as unemployment, poor living conditions, and discriminatory arrest practices.

Similar to these results for men, surveys (USDHHS, 1993) have suggested that African American women have similar drinking patterns to white women, but that African American women report higher abstention rates. For women, however, differences in alcohol-related problems were small, except drunk driving, which was reported more frequently by white females.

Hispanics. Hispanics in the United States, because of their cultural diversity, demonstrate variable drinking patterns. As in the general U.S. population, Hispanic men drink significantly more than Hispanic women and demonstrate concomitant alcohol-related problems. When compared to other racial and ethnic groups, Hispanic men have high rates of heavy drinking and a higher incidence of alcohol-related problems (Caetano, 1989). In a recent study of the effects of acculturation (the degree to which one adapts to and accepts cultural norms of a

new environment) on drinking practices, Caetano (1987) reported that more acculturated Hispanic men and women exhibited
drinking patterns closer to the general U.S. population. For
example, he found that highly acculturated Hispanic men (ages
40 and higher) and women (ages 18 and higher) showed lower
incidences of abstinence and higher rates of frequent heavy
drinking than those at lower acculturation levels.

Asian Americans. Asian American is a term encompassing a
diverse, rapidly growing segment of the U.S. population.
Although Asian American subgroups (e.g., populations with origins in Japan, China, Korea, India, and other Asian countries)
demonstrate varying alcohol use patterns, when taken as a
whole, Asian Americans exhibit the lowest level of alcohol consumption and related problems of all major racial and ethnic
groups in the United States (see reviews in USDHHS, 1990,
1993). These low rates of alcohol consumption and alcohol-
related problems have been attributed to sociocultural and environmental factors as well as to the alcohol-flush reaction. The
latter factor describes a physiological reaction to alcohol characterized by facial flushing, often with accompanying palpita-
tions, dizziness, nausea, and other symptoms of discomfort.
Although Asian Americans have shown low levels of drinking
and related problems, a review by Sue (1987) indicated that frequency and amount of drinking appeared to be increasing in
this population.

American Indian and Alaska Native Tribes. There are more than
300 American Indian and Alaska Native tribes in the United
States recognized by the federal government. These tribes represent an array of sociocultural customs (May, 1989). Drinking
patterns and alcohol-related problems among these tribes vary
considerably and therefore make it inappropriate to generalize
about alcohol use among this population. Despite high diversity in drinking practices across tribes, as a whole the American Indian and Native Alaskan population in 1988 experienced
an alcoholism death rate that was 5.4 times higher than the
U.S. alcoholism death rate for all races (Indian Health Service,
1991). Although a stereotype has suggested that "Indians cannot hold their liquor," evidence indicates that Indians do not
have innate physiological vulnerabilities that could explain the
high incidence of negative, alcohol-related consequences (May,
1989). Recent evidence has suggested that poverty and other

sociocultural factors may play an important causative role in Indian alcohol use (Adrian, Layne, & Williams, 1990–1991). Though the alcohol-related mortality rate among American Indians and Alaskan Natives remains critically high, prevention efforts developed by the Indian Health Services starting in 1986 have begun to show signs of positive impact on alcohol-related problems (Rhoades, Mason, Eddy, Smith, & Burns, 1988).

ECONOMIC COSTS OF ALCOHOL ABUSE

Alcohol use and abuse are associated with many costs to society both for drinkers and nondrinkers. For example, heavy drinking has been linked to adverse health consequences, which increase medical care costs and related insurance premiums. Alcohol consumption also has been associated with accidents and injuries, lost productivity in the workplace, criminal activity, and disturbances in family relationships. The total costs associated with alcohol abuse and dependence in the United States have been estimated at $98.6 billion for 1990 (Rice, 1993). Although this is a staggering sum of money, estimates and projections from earlier years have been even larger (see reviews in USDHHS, 1990, 1993), which indicates the inexact nature of these estimates. Despite their inaccuracies, however, these estimates provide valuable information about the magnitude of alcohol-related problems in the United States.

Other studies suggest that alcoholism treatment can be a wise investment, both from the standpoint of reducing human suffering and for economic reasons. For example, untreated alcoholics incur increasing health care costs in the years immediately preceding alcoholism treatment, which may reach as much as 300 percent higher immediately before treatment than nonalcoholics (Holder, 1987). Following treatment, however, declining trends in health care costs for alcoholics have been demonstrated for up to seven years (Blose & Holder, 1991). A more recent study (Holder & Blose, 1992), comparing health care expenditures of alcoholics treated for their alcoholism with untreated alcoholics, found that the former group incurred medical care costs that were 24 percent less than the latter over a four-year post-treatment period. Taken together the results of these studies suggest that providing alcohol treatment is a potentially successful method to reduce health care costs for alcoholics.

DIAGNOSIS OF ALCOHOL ABUSE AND DEPENDENCE

Methods used to diagnose alcohol-related disorders have evolved substantially in the last 25 years and have reflected the extant beliefs about the disorders. The American Psychiatric Association (APA) and the World Health Organization (WHO) have developed two of the more influential classification systems for substance-related disorders. These classification systems incorporate operational definitions as well as diagnostic criteria to identify alcohol-related disorders. Predating these efforts, the National Council on Alcoholism (NCA) spearheaded the first major attempt to diagnose alcoholism using definite criteria. The NCA criteria consisted of 86 physiological and clinical signs, and behavioral, psychological, and attitudinal symptoms (Babor, Kranzler, & Kadden, 1986). Although the NCA classification system was an important step developmentally, the system proved cumbersome, and attempts to test the criteria in clinical settings were unsuccessful (Jacobson, 1983).

The classification systems developed by the APA and the WHO have been modified frequently in the last 25 years. The latest edition of the APA's *Diagnostic and Statistical Manual of Mental Disorders* (*DSM-IV*) (American Psychiatric Association [APA], 1994) uses cognitive, behavioral, and physiological criteria for the diagnosis of substance dependence, including alcohol dependence (see table 1.1). Specifiers, indicating whether physiological dependence on alcohol exists, and course specifiers, describing conditions related to remission of symptoms, further delineate the diagnosis. Criteria for alcohol abuse focus on alcohol consumption that constitutes a maladaptive pattern of use associated with recurrent negative consequences (see table 1.2 for criteria used to diagnose alcohol and other substance abuse). The alcohol abuse diagnostic category is only used when the criteria for dependence have not previously been met. In other words, once an individual's drinking patterns and consequences have met the criteria for alcohol dependence, he or she may no longer be diagnosed as an alcohol abuser.

The WHO's *International Classification of Diseases* is currently in its 10th revision (*ICD-10*) (World Health Organization [WHO], 1992) and, like the *DSM-IV*, relies heavily on cognitive, behavioral, and physiological components for the diagnosis of alcohol dependence. Indeed, both diagnostic classification systems have

TABLE 1.1

Criteria for Substance Dependence

A maladaptive pattern of substance use, leading to clinically significant impairment or distress, as manifested by three (or more) of the following, occurring at any time in the same 12-month period:

1. Tolerance, as defined by either of the following
    a. A need for markedly increased amounts of the substance to achieve intoxication or desired effect
    b. Markedly diminished effect with continued use of the same amount of the substance
2. Withdrawal, as manifested by either of the following
    a. The characteristic withdrawal syndrome for the substance
    b. The same (or a closely related) substance is taken to relieve or avoid withdrawal symptoms
3. The substance is often taken in larger amounts or over a longer period than was intended
4. There is a persistent desire or there are unsuccessful efforts to cut down or control substance use
5. A great deal of time is spent in activities necessary to obtain the substance (e.g., visiting multiple doctors or driving long distances), use the substance (e.g., chain-smoking), or recover from its effects
6. Important social, occupational, or recreational activities are given up or reduced because of substance use
7. The substance use is continued despite knowledge of having a persistent or recurrent physical or psychological problem that is likely to have been caused or exacerbated by the substance (e.g., current cocaine use despite recognition of cocaine-induced depression, or continued drinking despite recognition that an ulcer was made worse by alcohol consumption)

Specifiers
>   With physiological dependence—evidence of tolerance or withdrawal (i.e., either item 1 or 2 is present)
>   Without physiological dependence—no evidence of tolerance or withdrawal (i.e., neither item 1 nor 2 is present)

Course specifiers
>   Early full remission
>   Early partial remission
>   Sustained full remission
>   Sustained partial remission
>   On agonist therapy
>   In a controlled environment

Adapted with permission from the Diagnostic and Statistical Manual of Mental Disorders, Fourth Edition, Washington D.C. American Psychiatric Association, 1994.

TABLE 1.2

Criteria for Substance Abuse

A. A maladaptive pattern of substance use leading to clinically significant impairment or distress, as manifested by one (or more) of the following, occurring within a 12-month period:
  1. Recurrent substance use resulting in a failure to fulfill major role obligations at work, school, or home (e.g., repeated absences or poor work performance related to substance use; substance-related absences, suspensions, or expulsions from school; neglect of children or household)
  2. Recurrent substance use in situations in which it is physically hazardous (e.g., driving an automobile or operating a machine when impaired by substance use)
  3. Recurrent substance-related legal problems (e.g., arrests for substance-related disorderly conduct)
  4. Continued substance use despite having persistent or recurrent social or interpersonal problems caused or exacerbated by the effects of the substance (e.g., arguments with spouse about consequences of intoxication, physical fights)
B. The symptoms have never met the criteria for substance dependence for this class of substance.

Adapted with permission from The Diagnostic and Statistical Manual of Mental Disorders, Fourth Edition. Washington D.C. American Psychiatric Association, 1994.

historical roots in the alcohol dependence syndrome described by Edwards and Gross (1976). Although some differences remain in the two systems, these latest revisions represent closer agreement. Both systems characterize alcohol dependence similarly, based on detailed multiple criteria for alcohol-related disorders. Both also have a category describing consumption that is harm producing but does not meet criteria for alcohol dependence. For a more detailed discussion of the evolution of the diagnostic criteria used in the APA and the WHO classification systems, see the *Eighth Special Report to the U.S. Congress on Alcohol and Health* (USDHHS, 1993).

ALCOHOL ABUSE AND DEPENDENCE AND ASSOCIATED MEDICAL AND PSYCHIATRIC MORBIDITY AND MORTALITY

Although U.S. per capita alcohol consumption has been steadily declining in recent years, overall alcohol-related morbidity

13

(measured by short-stay community hospital discharges) remained relatively constant from 1979 to 1993 (Fe Caces, Stinson, & Dufour, 1995). Recent studies have estimated the incidence of alcohol-related problems among hospitalized persons to be 22 percent (Umbricht-Schneiter, Santora, & Moore, 1991) and 25 percent (Moore et al., 1989). However, these percentages will vary across hospital departments and will depend on the skill and vigilance of staff in identifying patients with alcohol problems. Unfortunately, there is evidence to indicate that physicians often underdiagnose alcohol abuse and dependence (Moore et al., 1989), which suggests that alcohol-related morbidity may be underestimated. Underdiagnosis was most frequent on surgical and obstetrics-gynecology departments in the Moore et al. study.

Alcohol use has been documented as a significant contributor to mortality in the United States and may be underestimated due to the underreporting of the incidence of alcohol-related deaths. A recent study of the major external (nongenetic) factors contributing to death in the United States in 1990 indicated that alcohol use was ranked as the third leading contributor to death, behind tobacco use and diet and activity patterns (McGinnis & Foege, 1993). Cirrhosis of the liver, a significant health hazard associated with alcohol use, was the ninth leading cause of death in the U.S. in 1988 (Grant, DeBakey, & Zobeck, 1991). It has maintained this significant position despite substantial declines in cirrhosis mortality rates since a peak was reached in 1973, when the age-adjusted death rate for cirrhosis was 14.9 deaths per 100,000 population. In 1992, the age-adjusted rate was 8.1 deaths per 100,000 population, representing a 45.6 percent reduction since 1973 (DeBakey, Stinson, Grant, & Dufour, 1995).

Alcohol-Related Psychiatric Morbidity and Mortality

Along with the negative effects of alcohol abuse on the body, it has become progressively apparent in recent years that alcohol abuse and dependence are often associated with psychiatric comorbidities, including the abuse of other drugs. An extensive survey of psychiatric disorders in the general population (Helzer & Pryzbeck, 1988) found that about 14 percent of those surveyed reported lifetime prevalence of alcohol abuse or dependence, with approximately half of this group reporting another psychiatric diagnosis. The diagnosis of alcohol dependence was five times more prevalent in men than women. However, alcohol dependence was more strongly associated with other diagnoses in women: 65 percent of alcohol-dependent women had a second diagnosis, compared with 44 percent of alcohol-dependent men; 31 percent of alcohol-dependent women had a diagnosis of drug abuse or dependence, whereas 19 percent of alcohol-dependent men had one of these two diagnoses. When compared with men and women in the general population, alcohol-dependent men and women have higher prevalence rates for antisocial personality disorder and major depression. Although the Helzer and Pryzbeck study was plagued by methodological problems resulting in prevalence overestimates in some disorders, it gives an overview of the high incidence of co-occurring psychiatric disorders among alcohol abusers.

Psychiatric Comorbidity Among Patients in Treatment for Alcohol Abuse or Dependence

A high incidence of co-occurring psychiatric disorders is characteristic of patients in treatment for alcohol or drug problems as well. In a survey of patients seeking assistance for alcohol and drug problems, Ross, Glaser, and Germanson (1988) found that 78 percent of this population reported a history of psychiatric disorder in addition to substance abuse, and approximately 65 percent had a current psychiatric disorder. This study also found that patients abusing both alcohol and drugs demonstrated the most psychiatric impairment, which is a finding that recent research supports (O'Boyle, 1993).

A major issue in treating patients with psychiatric problems co-occurring with alcohol abuse is discriminating psychopathology that is nonalcohol related from symptoms of transient states of alcohol withdrawal or intoxication (Blankfield, 1986). Symptoms such as anxiety and depression are common in patients withdrawing from alcohol and do not necessarily indicate independent anxiety or mood disorders. As the patient progresses through withdrawal, these symptoms often resolve themselves without additional treatment.

Although most alcoholics entering treatment do not demonstrate deficits in overall intellectual functioning, a majority have deficits in problem solving, nonverbal abstract reasoning, concept shifting, psychomotor skills, and certain memory tasks (Eckardt & Martin, 1986; Parsons & Leber, 1981; Tabakoff &

Petersen, 1988). These deficits typically improve with continued abstinence and often resolve completely over time. However, treatment professionals must consider that alcoholics frequently enter rehabilitative programs with cognitive deficits that may interfere with their ability to learn informational content, particularly during the first 2 weeks of care (Goldman, 1986). We must consider these cognitive deficits and modify treatment approaches as necessary for successful outcome (Goldman, 1987).

As indicated by a recent review (USDHHS, 1993), co-occurring alcohol-related and other psychiatric disorders adversely affect the clinical course of both disorders and present significant challenges to treatment professionals. In addition, traditional treatment approaches for alcohol-related disorders have been relatively ineffective with patients having co-occurring disorders (McLellan, Erdlen, Erdlen, & O'Brien, 1981). Therefore, to be successful, future treatment efforts should address the unique needs of this population (USDHHS, 1993).

THEORIES OF ETIOLOGY AND DEVELOPMENT OF ALCOHOL DEPENDENCE

There are many theories attempting to explain alcohol dependence. These theories reflect the field that their proponents represent. Therefore, there are theories originating in the biological sciences that suggest genetic and biological substrates that account for individuals developing alcohol dependence. There are theories relying on psychological factors as most influential in the etiology of alcohol dependence. Finally, there are theories proposing that social variables account for the etiology of alcohol dependence. As Cahalan (1988) suggested, there is a great deal of "reductionist chauvinism" (p. xxiv) in the field of alcohol studies, which has led to isolated theory development and few attempts to integrate developments across disciplines. Cahalan further indicated that this theoretical isolationism is from theorists being mesmerized with their own work, as well as scientists and practitioners lacking breadth of background to fully appreciate the complex nature of alcohol dependence. Realizing that none of the individual theories will sufficiently account for the etiology and development of alcohol dependence, the following descriptions provide the reader with some basis for understanding this multifaceted problem.

Biological Theories

Theories subsumed under the rubric *biological* assert that alcohol dependence is predominately determined by genetically transmitted characteristics. Therefore, biological theories suggest that genetic inheritance determines an individual's risk for alcohol dependence. Studies on the familial incidence of alcohol dependence, concordance rates for alcohol dependence between twins, and studies of the effects of adoption and environment on development of alcohol dependence add to the notion that, in some circumstances, alcohol dependence may be related to genetically determined predisposing factors. Although questions remain regarding the methodology and conclusions drawn from these studies (Lester, 1988), biological predisposing factors appear to play a role in the etiology of alcohol dependence.

Exactly what is inherited or genetically transmitted that predisposes one to alcohol dependence? It is likely that the development of alcohol dependence involves not one but a constellation of genes that play a role in predisposing the individual. Tabakoff and Hoffman (1988), in their explication of a neurobiological theory of alcohol dependence, suggest that what is genetically transmitted is a "sensitivity to the aversive and reinforcing affects of ethanol" (p. 33), which predisposes the individual to alcohol abuse and dependence. More specifically, Tabakoff and Hoffman suggested that the individual prone to alcohol dependence is genetically predisposed to develop tolerance to the aversive effects of alcohol (e.g., central nervous system depressant effects), which allows the positively reinforcing effects of alcohol (e.g., decreased inhibitions) to predominate.

What is genetically transmitted to predispose the individual to alcohol dependence in an alternative way? The neurobehavioral theory of the etiology of alcohol dependence, as proposed by Tarter, Alterman, and Edwards (1988), suggests that certain behavioral disturbances that create a susceptibility to alcohol dependence are inherited. They have suggested that these disturbances include lack of emotional control (lability), impersistence, disinhibition, hyperactivity, attention deficits, and cognitive impairments frequently found in persons with lesions in the anterior-basal brain region. Although the theory focuses on characteristic behavioral disturbances that may play an etiological role in developing alcohol dependence, it also relates these behavioral variables to underlying neurochemical and neurophysiological processes, and finally to a specific neuroanatomical substrate. Therefore, the theory conceptualizes vulnerability to alcohol dependence as a result of multilevel disturbances that yield maladaptive psychological functioning. The theory is in a stage of infancy; however, it should serve to stimulate further investigation of other behavioral precursors of alcohol dependence.

Psychological Theories

A second subset of theories regarding alcohol abuse and dependence focuses on psychological factors. Theories reporting psychological causes of alcohol dependence are numerous and a detailed discussion of each is beyond the scope of this section. I refer the interested reader to a book edited by Blane and Leonard (1987) called *Psychological Theories of Drinking and Alcoholism*, the primary source for the summaries to follow.

Psychological theories of alcohol use have sought to explain initiation of drinking as well as transitions to other drinking statuses such as abuse and dependence. Historically, psychological theories have focused on alcohol as a tension reducer (tension reduction theory), on personality factors that may potentially make one more susceptible to drinking problems or be a result of heavy drinking (personality theory), on alcohol as a method of coping with everyday life demands (social learning theory), and on the complex interaction between person and environmental variables, particularly during adolescence, that lead to initiation of alcohol use and possibly to problem drinking (interactional theory). These four theoretical groupings represent traditional approaches to explaining alcohol use and abuse through psychological mechanisms. More recently, other theoretical models have surfaced that either are related to or are outgrowths from the longer-standing traditional approaches.

Alcohol-Related Expectancies. Expectancy theory, developmentally related to social learning theory, is an example of a more recent model to explain alcohol use and abuse. This theory asserts that an individual's expectation of the effects of alcohol plays an important role in the initiation of alcohol use, maintenance of use, increased alcohol use in some individuals, and continued use despite negative consequences in the alcohol abuser and alcoholic. This theory has been instrumental in increasing our understanding of the crucial role that expectancies play in the development of alcohol dependence as well as the recovery process.

Stress Response Dampening. Closely related to the tension reduction theory, stress response dampening focuses on the ability of alcohol to *dampen* the physiologic response to stress. This subjective alleviation of the body's response to stress reinforces drinking and enhances the probability that drinking will occur in similar situations in the future. Although the stress response dampening model focuses on pharmacologic effects of alcohol, it also recognizes the important role of expectancies and individual differences in sensitivity to the stress dampening response as determinants of alcohol use.

Self-Awareness. The self-awareness model is similar to the stress response dampening model in that it relies on alcohol's pharmacologic properties to explain causes and effects of alcohol use. This theory suggests that alcohol decreases self-awareness, therefore leading to a decrease in appropriate behavior (i.e., behavioral disinhibition) and a decrease in negative self-evaluation following failure, which is sufficient to precipitate and sustain drinking. Although this theory is limited in its explanatory value, it explains drinking in situations that may have particular relevance to the sport world. Sport has many situations in which negative self-evaluations occur (e.g., following a disappointing performance), which may invite heavy drinking to reduce this negative affective state.

Self-Handicapping. Self-handicapping theory also has direct relevance to the sport world. Self-handicapping involves individuals using a tactic to provide them with protection for a positive competence image through controlling attributions for their behavior. Using alcohol before performance evaluations is one example of a self-handicapping tactic. The individual can attribute failure under the influence of alcohol to the effects of alcohol and not to lack of competence. If a person achieves success under these circumstances, competence image is enhanced because success was achieved despite the negative influence of alcohol. This theory may provide a basis for understanding abusive drinking in individuals characterized as successful, including athletes.

Opponent Processes. This psychologically based theory focuses on the apparent *opponent processes* that occur during and following drinking. The theory holds that drinking alcohol results in direct physiologic effects counteracted by a rebound effect when an individual stops drinking. For example, drinking initially may result in pleasant, euphoric effects followed by an overcorrecting rebound the next morning (hangover). According to the theory, as drinking continues, the rebound mechanism becomes stronger through repetition, therefore reducing the immediate pleasurable effect of alcohol and requiring more alcohol than previously needed to achieve the same effect (i.e., tolerance). Addiction occurs as the individual continues to drink to alleviate this increasing rebound mechanism that is experienced as a negative state (i.e., withdrawal).

Social Theories

Theories purporting social explanations for alcohol use and abuse emanate from the fields of sociology, anthropology, and economics. A sociocultural model, deriving mostly from sociology and anthropology, suggests that the frequency in which alcohol problems occur across cultures, as well as the differences in the nature of these problems, is a product of variable beliefs and attitudes about alcohol and its effects, along with societal rules regarding drinking situations. In particular, these rules are prescriptions and proscriptions concerning when, where, how, and with whom one should or should not drink (Heath, 1988). Although the sociocultural model takes various forms and is supported by various research paradigms, its impact on the field has been profound. As noted by Heath (1988), we can make several important conclusions about alcohol use based on the sociocultural perspective:

1. Drinking is a social act that people are rarely neutral about.
2. Norms regarding drinking are emotionally charged and include expectations about the effects of drinking.
3. Drunken behavior conforms to prescriptive patterns and is affected by social learning.
4. In most cultures where drinking occurs, alcohol-related problems are infrequent and addiction is rare on a worldwide basis.
5. The cultural context often plays a major role in the cause of drinking problems that occur in the individual living in the culture.
6. There is no cross culturally consistent development of alcohol-related problems or ways in which they are manifested.

Availability theory of alcohol-related problems is another of the social theories (Single, 1988). Its basic premise is that the prevalence and severity of alcohol-related problems directly relate to the availability of alcohol in a particular society or culture. Alcohol availability refers to both physical accessibility (e.g., number of retail outlets, purchase restrictions) and economic accessibility (e.g., price and affordability to the consumer). This theory would suggest that limiting availability of alcohol will reduce the incidence of alcohol-related problems. These problems include those associated with alcohol dependence such as cirrhosis, and other problems not necessarily associated with alcohol dependence, including alcohol-related violence, drinking and driving, and low productivity in the workforce. Because there has been an increase in alcohol consumption, along with increases in alcohol-related health and social problems in the industrialized world since World War II, there has been increased attention on controls over alcohol availability as a prevention for alcohol-related problems. In addition to controls on alcohol accessibility, control methods have been considered for advertising alcoholic beverages. Because the alcohol industry supports many athletic events through advertising funds, this prevention method, if implemented, may have significant effects on the sport world.

As we can see from these theories accounting for alcohol abuse and dependence, the alcohol field does not lack theoretical foundation. A commonly held belief is that alcohol dependence is a biopsychosocial problem or disease. As suggested by Cahalan (1988), what we need now is to focus on how we can integrate these theories to provide a more comprehensive explanation for etiology of alcohol dependence. This integration will require cross-disciplinary communication and investigation.

RISK FACTORS FOR ALCOHOL DEPENDENCE

Numerous risk factors have been associated with developing alcohol dependence; however, the most powerful predictor appears to be a family history of alcohol dependence (Tarter & Edwards, 1986). Although recent evidence suggests that alcohol dependence is in part caused by genetic transmission, as indicated in the section on biological theories, the question of what exactly is inherited remains unanswered. What we know at this point is that the development of alcohol dependence is a complicated process, including risk factors associated not only with an individual's biological makeup but also with psychological constitution and social environment. This spectrum of potential risk factors is exemplified in a recent review of factors that place youth at risk for alcohol and other drug use, abuse, or dependence (Lorion, Bussell, & Goldberg, 1991). These factors included variables related to economic disadvantage; race or ethnicity; family of origin; peer groups; gender; age; behavioral symptoms such as antisocial behaviors; school and learning problems; attitudes and beliefs about alcohol and other drug use; and personality characteristics such as rebelliousness, alienation, a strong need for independence, and a high tolerance for deviance. Further, it appears that particular risk factors become more pronounced and operative at various times in the addictive cycle. For instance, social factors are quite influential in the initiation of alcohol use, and physical and psychological factors increase in prominence as the addiction process continues (Lettieri, 1987).

Because individuals may express biological and psychological vulnerabilities to alcohol dependence behaviorally, researchers have pursued behavioral indicants associated with developing alcohol dependence. For instance, research has found that childhood conduct disorder and hyperactivity frequently predate alcohol dependence and may constitute, along with other childhood behavioral disturbances and adult psychopathology, psychological vulnerabilities to alcohol dependence (Alterman & Tarter, 1983). Related research reviewed by Tarter (1985) suggests that a disturbed central nervous system underlies these behavioral problems, along with other problems that predate alcohol dependence. A frequent behavioral pattern for a prealcoholic individual is impulsivity, poor self-control, and aggressiveness. These traits are often associated with antisocial proclivities, which are in turn associated with increased risk for alcohol dependence.

More recent research has supported the notion that behavioral symptom clusters may predate and occur concurrently with the development of alcohol dependence. A recent prospective study (Andréasson, Allebeck, & Brandt, 1993) in Sweden indicated that poor emotional control and early symptoms of mental disorder were associated with risk for high consumption of alcohol and ensuing risk for developing alcohol abuse and dependence in Swedish male military conscripts. Another study on psychiatric disorders in adult children of alcoholics (Mathew,

Wilson, Blazer, & George, 1993) found that these individuals experienced significantly higher prevalence rates of various psychiatric disorders, such as simple phobia, dysthymia (depressive symptoms), generalized anxiety disorder, panic disorder, and antisocial symptoms, than a matched control group of subjects who did not have one or more alcoholic parents. This study suggests that individuals with a family history of alcohol dependence are not only at risk for developing alcohol problems but also at risk for other psychiatric disorders. Depending on when they become apparent, these psychiatric symptoms may be a useful marker to identify individuals who are at increased risk for alcohol dependence.

At present our ability to predict who will develop problems with alcohol, including alcohol abuse and dependence, is not well honed. There appear to be numerous correlates of alcohol dependence that may precede its development and therefore be of value in identifying at-risk individuals. We have strong evidence that those with a family history of alcohol dependence are at increased risk, but we don't understand the mechanisms that underlie this risk. Therefore, at best we can speculate about a composite picture of those individuals at higher risk for alcohol dependence. This composite description might include an individual who has a family history of alcohol dependence, who may or may not have experienced related psychiatric symptoms, such as childhood conduct disorder, hyperactivity, antisocial behavior (e.g., truancy, authority problems), generalized anxiety, and use of other drugs besides alcohol. There is also indication that this composite may differ by gender, with males demonstrating higher rates of antisocial symptoms and abuse of other drugs and females showing higher rates of generalized anxiety (Mathew, Wilson, Blazer, & George, 1993). In addition to these biological and psychological characteristics, the at-risk individual may experience social factors that promote alcohol use, such as easy access to alcohol and membership in a culture or peer group that values alcohol consumption. Keeping these biopsychosocial risk factors in mind, it is possible to make reasonable assumptions about an individual's risk for alcoholism.

CONCLUSION

Alcohol use is a part of many persons' lifestyles in the United States. Epidemiological data indicate that alcohol use starts during adolescence for most drinkers and occurs, in varying levels of frequency and intensity, across gender, race, and ethnic origin. Although a small minority of adults meet diagnostic criteria for alcohol abuse or dependence, many drinkers experience alcohol-related problems. Risk factors for alcohol dependence have been identified (a family history of alcohol dependence being the strongest); however, our ability to predict who will become dependent on alcohol is limited. Costs (economic and otherwise) of alcohol abuse and dependence are staggering; however, treatment has shown promise in decreasing the health care expenditures of alcoholics.

In this chapter we have focused on general information regarding alcohol and addiction. In chapter 2, we will discuss how alcohol relates to sport in the United States. Please keep in mind what you have learned in this chapter, as this knowledge will give you the background to evaluate information in chapter 2 as well as ensuing chapters.

2 ALCOHOL USE IN SPORT

What is going on when Americans insist on immersing wholesome sport in a sea of intoxicating drink?

—W. Johnson

We will now turn our attention to the relationship of alcohol use and sport. In chapter 2, we first explore factors that have contributed to a symbiosis between beer breweries and sport. In this context, we will discuss the foundations of the relationship between the beer industry and sport teams and the consequences of this relationship. The balance of the chapter discusses alcohol use in the general population and among athletes, sport professionals, and sport spectators. The section on alcohol use in the general population provides some basis for comparing alcohol use in sport-related populations. We hope that the reader will glean from this chapter an understanding of the level of alcohol use among sport-related populations and of the market forces that promote alcohol use in the sport context.

ASSOCIATION OF ALCOHOL AND SPORT IN THE UNITED STATES

The association of alcohol and sport has a storied past and may have some distant roots in the competition of war. Commenting on the importance of beer to his soldiers, in 1777, Frederick the Great, King of Prussia, said:

> *My people must drink beer. His majesty was brought up on beer and so were his officers and soldiers. Many battles have been fought and won by soldiers nourished on beer, and the King does not believe that coffee-drinking soldiers can be depended on to endure hardships or to beat the enemies. (Johnson, 1988, p. 71)*

Certainly this love of alcoholic beverages is not lost on soldiers in the time of Frederick the Great. Drinking continues to occupy a significant role in the modern military and often serves as the focus of social gatherings as well as the source of problems.

Just as in the military, alcohol, in particular beer, has played a significant role in sport. From the club rugby teams where beer drinking is an assumed after-game activity to an afternoon at the baseball park, consuming alcoholic beverages is a high-profile activity in sport. As Johnson suggested in "Sports and Suds," his 1988 *Sports Illustrated* article, "beer and sport have come to be as inseparable in the American lexicon as mom and apple pie, God and country, ham and eggs, Jack and Jill and, of course, suds and Spuds" (p. 70). This strong attachment between beer and sport is not limited to the United States, but characterizes other countries as well. For example, soccer fans in western European countries often consume large quantities of beer and other alcoholic beverages. Crawford (1977) described the relationship of alcohol and sport clubs in New Zealand, noting concern that sport clubs may become de facto taverns because many have been granted ancillary liquor licenses.

Literature and film also have depicted the alcohol and sport connection. Ardolino (1991) analyzed novels and films that have included a connection between bars and sport. For example, he discusses the role that Andy's Italian-American Bar plays in the film *Rocky*, the story of an unknown Italian-American boxer who gets his chance to fight the heavyweight champion. Ardolino suggested that in various ways bars have been used to develop stories in literature and in film about sport figures.

Duplicate Demographics and the Profit Motive

How is it that sport, an activity intended to produce healthy minds and bodies, is juxtaposed with beer, a potentially addictive substance with few, if any, redeeming health values? The answer appears to be that the demographics of beer drinkers and sport fans are largely synonymous. "Beer drinkers and sports fans are one and the same—indivisible, inseparable, identical! No one drinks more beer than a sports fan, and no one likes sports more than a beer drinker" (Johnson, 1988, p. 74). Although this quotation may exaggerate to make a point, realizing the significance of this relationship between sport and beer drinking, August A. Busch, Jr., president of the Anheuser-Busch brewery, helped to solidify this demographic relationship when he purchased the St. Louis Cardinals in 1953. With this purchase, Mr. Busch strengthened the relationship between beer and baseball by recognizing the potential profitability of the partnership for both parties. From 1953 to 1978, Anheuser-Busch brewery annual sales grew from less than 6 million to more than 35 million barrels. In an interview in *The Sporting News* in 1978, Mr. Busch attributed this growth partly to the company's association with baseball (Johnson, 1988).

Realizing the potential of an affiliation with sport, Anheuser-Busch and Miller breweries began to spend enormous sums of money for sport-related advertising during the 1970s. The competition between the two breweries for advertising and sponsorship rights in sport has continued ever since. In 1988, Anheuser-Busch spent two-thirds of its $344 million advertising budget in sport-related areas, and from 1977 to 1988 the company's share of the national beer market jumped from 22 percent to 40 percent (Johnson, 1988). Anheuser-Busch and Miller have dominated advertising on network television during the last 15 years, primarily through exclusivity clauses that make it difficult for other breweries to advertise through this medium.

Anheuser-Busch also has dominated sponsorship of professional and amateur sport teams and events, whereby they support a team or event in return for agreements on product promotions. In 1991, Anheuser-Busch helped support all Major League Baseball teams, 20 of 28 National Football League teams, more than 300 college teams, and approximately 1,000 other sporting events, such as triathlons, skiing, and cycling races (Nelson, 1991).

What has developed between breweries and sport, particularly during the last 20 years, is a tightly woven symbiotic relationship. The beer industry is keenly aware that its advertising dollars are best spent in sport, where many of the industry's most loyal customers lie. On the other hand, the sport world is heavily dependent on the advertising revenue generated by the beer companies, which permits sporting events and leagues to survive whereas otherwise they might be financially insolvent. This is most true in amateur sport. For example, one of Miller brewery's contracts from 1981 to 1988 was a $1 million-a-year commitment for operating expenses for the U.S. Olympic Committee's training facilities. Labatt Brewing Company in Toronto has been a major contributor to the Olympics in Canada. The company was a sponsor of the 1988 Winter Games in Calgary, contributing approximately $25 million Canadian (Johnson, 1988).

The major breweries have significant presence in the motor sports as well, particularly as sponsors. A report sponsored by AAA Foundation for Traffic Safety (Buchanan & Lev, 1989) indicated that motor sport fans, composed largely of blue collar male youth and young adults, are heavy beer drinkers, and therefore are a target population for breweries. These researchers studied beer industry expenditures and justifications for sport-related sponsorships during 1989. They found that (a) brewers are second only to tobacco industry sponsors in dollars spent, (b) sport receives the largest share of dollars spent for sponsorship, and (c) motor sports lead all other sports in the amount of sponsorship money they receive.

Breweries' underwriting of motor sports is an example of the target marketing that has characterized the industry since Phillip Morris, the cigarette manufacturer, purchased Miller Brewing Company in 1970. Along with this purchase came the marketing strategies honed in the cigarette industry, which include target marketing and image-oriented selling. The primary goal of these marketing strategies is to identify the segments of the population that are most likely to purchase the product and target the advertising message to that subpopulation. Various sports offer natural avenues for industry marketers to reach their target populations. As suggested in a recent *USA Today* article (Hiestand, 1993), targeting demographics will likely be a dominant strategy in the future for television networks. Networks will show sports that can provide the right kind of demographics to the potential advertiser. An often coveted demographic group in this marketing strategy is young people, partly because they have yet to establish brand loyalties.

This type of demographic-driven sales, along with escalating finances associated with sport (e.g., professional players' salaries, television rights), will most likely continue to solidify the relationship between beer and sport because the advertising dollars will be valued even more. Those sports not able to provide the necessary demographics to advertisers will likely be in financial trouble. For example, there has been concern expressed in baseball management that their fan base is aging. Therefore baseball will become less attractive to advertisers, particularly the beer industry, because young males consume most of the beer (Greising, 1993).

Alcohol Advertising and Sponsorship: Population Effects

An important question asked with more frequency since the sport and beer advertising relationship has developed is, what message does this relationship send to the general population, in particular youth, who are forming important attitudes and behaviors that will extend into adulthood? An analysis of beer commercials completed under the auspices of the AAA Foundation for Traffic Safety by Postman, Nystrom, Strate, and Weingartner (1987) provides some information regarding this question. They found that between the ages of 2 and 18, American children see approximately 100,000 commercials for beer on television. This developmental period is also characterized by social learning in which the child acquires knowledge and skills she or he will carry into later life stages. Of interest to these researchers were the general themes of the commercials and how association of these themes promoted beer. They found that the predominant theme in beer commercials was masculinity. The researchers indicated that through exposure to typical beer commercials, the viewer was given a selective stereotype of manhood. They found "no sensitive men in beer commercials—nor any thoughtful men, scholarly men, political men, gay men, or even complex men" (Postman et al., p. 47). The researchers indicated that commercials typically portray men as active in work and play and prone to seek activities characterized by physical challenge, risk taking, and danger. Comparatively, "women are reduced largely to the role of admiring onlookers. . . . They become the audience for whom men perform" (Postman et al., p. 44). In sum, they described the stereotype of both men and women to be "laughably anachronistic . . . a peculiar set of figures to offer the young of the 1980's as models of adult females and males" (Postman et al., p. 48).

Of further importance in this study is that, almost without exception, the commercials presented beer drinking as an essential ingredient of masculinity. They promoted the idea that to be regarded as a real man in American culture and be accepted by peers, one must drink beer. Finally, and perhaps of most concern to the physical safety of potential beer consumers and others, these researchers concluded that beer commercials frequently promote the association, albeit implicit, of beer drinking and driving. The final recommendation of the researchers is that policies allowing beer advertising on television be altered to prohibit such commercials.

These results suggest that alcohol advertising may have detrimental effects on the alcohol-related attitudes and practices of the general population; however, evidence for these effects is lacking (Partanen & Montonen, 1988; Sobell et al., 1986). This lack of evidence of detrimental effects combined with the large financial incentives for alcohol advertising make it difficult to imagine that significant changes will occur in advertising practices in the near future. Stricter forms of regulation have been entertained, such as a ban on *lifestyle* advertising and a ban on alcohol advertising in the broadcast media. However, these proposed bans would rely on popular support based on public concern about ill effects of alcohol on society at large. Whether this support is present or forthcoming is yet to be seen. Education as opposed to censorship is an alternative method of altering the potential negative effects of alcohol advertising. Chapter 5 will discuss promising educational methods.

ALCOHOL USE IN THE GENERAL POPULATION

Drinking alcoholic beverages is a commonplace activity in the United States as well as in most other Western cultures. When considering the significance of alcohol use among any subpopulation, such as athletes or sport professionals, it is important to look at the drinking incidence and consequences in the cultural context. Recent data from the *National Household Survey on Drug Abuse* (Substance Abuse and Mental Health Services Administration [SAMHSA], 1995) indicated that alcohol remained the overwhelming drug of choice in the United States when compared with nicotine (in cigarettes and smokeless tobacco) and illicit drugs (e.g., marijuana, cocaine). This survey was completed with U.S. population samples (a total of 26,489 respondents) and was designed to draw conclusions about the drug use of the civilian, noninstitutionalized population aged 12 and older (target population). The survey found that 84 percent of the target population reported lifetime use of alcohol, 67 percent reported use in the past year, and 50 percent reported use in the past month. The reported incidence of other drug use was vastly less than alcohol (see table 2.1).

When examining alcohol use across the life span, data suggest that use frequently begins in the early teen years, peaks in young adulthood, and decreases in middle to late adult years. In their recent survey results of secondary and collegiate students, Johnston, O'Malley, and Bachman (1995, 1996) reported that alcohol use is typical in this population. They reported lifetime use rates of 56 percent for 8th graders, 71 percent for 10th graders, 80 percent for 12th graders, and 88 percent for college students. Of additional concern is the widespread occurrence of reported heavy drinking (measured by the percentage reporting five or more drinks in a row at least once in the prior two weeks). For 8th graders this statistic was 15 percent, for 10th graders 24 percent, for 12th graders 28 percent, and for college students 40 percent. Following the early 20s, this percentage falls to 34 percent for the entire young adult sample (up to age 32). Although these rates of drinking may seem high, some good news is that current and heavy drinking rates among high school seniors, measured

TABLE 2.1

Percentage and Estimated Number of Users (in Thousands) of Illicit Drugs, Alcohol, and Tobacco in the U.S. Civilian, Noninstitutionalized Population Age 12 and Older in Their Lifetime, the Past Year, and the Past Month: 1993 (n = 26,489)

		TIME PERIOD				
	Lifetime		*Past year*		*Past month*	
Drug	%	Number of users (thousands)	%	Number of users (thousands)	%	Number of users (thousands)
Any illicit drug use[1]	37.2	77,022	11.8	24,437	5.6	11,705
Marijuana or hashish	33.7	69,923	9.0	18,573	4.3	8,992
Cocaine	11.3	23,494	2.2	4,530	0.6	1,307
Crack	1.8	3,749	0.5	996	0.2	417
Inhalants	5.3	10,900	1.0	2,092	0.4	889
Hallucinogens	8.7	18,054	1.2	2,391	0.2	515
PCP	4.1	8,412	0.2	448	0.1	155
Heroin	1.1	2,292	0.1	245	*	80
Nonmedical use of any psycho-therapeutic[2]	11.1	23,034	3.8	7,892	1.3	2,655
Stimulants	6.0	12,524	1.1	2,377	0.3	719
Sedatives	3.4	7,127	0.8	1,582	0.3	528
Tranquilizers	4.6	9,457	1.2	2,543	0.3	572
Analgesics	5.8	11,921	2.2	4,571	0.7	1,417
Alcohol	83.6	173,304	66.5	137,772	49.6	102,810
Cigarettes	71.2	147,519	29.4	60,966	24.2	50,114
Smokeless tobacco	12.8	26,493	4.0	8,243	2.9	6,095

* Low precision; no estimate reported.

[1] Use of marijuana or hashish, cocaine (including crack), inhalants, hallucinogens (including PCP), heroin, or nonmedical use of psychotherapeutics at least once.

[2] Nonmedical use of any prescription-type stimulant, sedative, tranquilizer, or analgesic; does not include over-the-counter drugs.

Note. From *National Household Survey on Drug Abuse: Main Findings 1993* (p. 24) by the Substance Abuse and Mental Health Services Administration, 1995, Rockville, MD: Author.

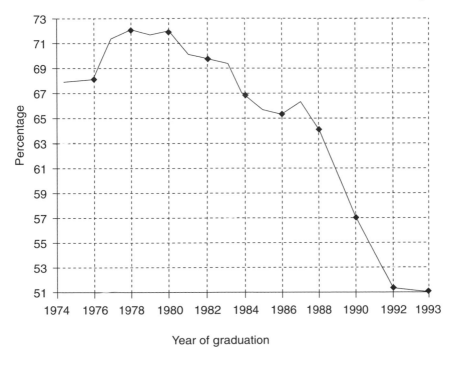

Figure 2.1 Percentage of high school seniors who were current drinkers (used alcohol in the past 30 days).

From *National Survey Results on Drug Use from the Monitoring the Future Study, 1975–1994: Volume 1. Secondary School Students* (p. 81) by L.D. Johnston, P.M. O'Malley, and J.G. Bachman, 1995, Washington, DC: U.S Government Printing Office.

by survey data, have trended downward since 1980 (see figures 2.1 and 2.2). This downward trend has paralleled a similar trend in use of many other drugs; however, reported illicit drug use increased in 1993 (Johnston, O'Malley, & Bachman, 1994) and 1994 (Johnston et al., 1995).

The decreasing trend in alcohol use by youth is positive; however, alcohol use by young people remains at a level warranting concern. In 1992, 8th graders were the only group that did not show a significant decline from 1991 in prevalence of drinking in the prior 30 days. There were declines, though not significant, in the daily drinking rates for 10th and 12th graders but not for the 8th-grade population. Eighth graders showed increases in both of these measures, though they were not statistically significant (Johnston, O'Malley, & Bachman, 1993).

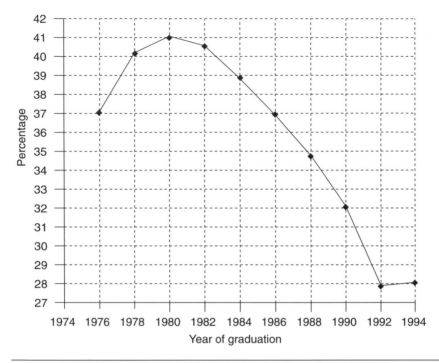

Figure 2.2 Percentage of high school seniors who were occasional heavy drinkers (took five or more drinks at least once in the past two weeks).

From *National Survey Results on Drug Use from the Monitoring the Future Study, 1975–1994: Volume 1. Secondary School Students* (p. 82) by L.D. Johnston, P.M. O'Malley, and J.G. Bachman, 1995, Washington, DC: U.S Government Printing Office.

Furthermore, in 1993, 26 percent of 8th graders reported already having been drunk at least once (Johnston et al., 1994). The large number of 8th graders that have already begun using alcohol as well as other drugs (tobacco, marijuana, inhalants— often referred to as gateway drugs because they precede the use of other drugs of abuse) suggests that many are already at risk for proceeding to other drugs such as LSD, cocaine, and amphetamines (Johnston et al., 1994).

Drinking incidence during the transition years from adolescence to young adulthood appears to be similar to high school seniors, with somewhat higher levels of daily drinking and of drinking within the preceding month (Johnston et al., 1995,

1996). However, there appears to be little continuity in drinking behavior from adolescence to young adulthood such that drinking behavior at age 18 is not a reliable predictor of drinking at age 25 or 30. Generally, however, aggregate data indicate that both current and heavier drinking become more likely between the ages of 17 and 22 and less likely through young adulthood for both sexes (see review in USDHHS, 1990).

Though there is inconsistency in results across longitudinal and cross-sectional studies examining the relationship of age to alcohol use, generally alcohol consumption remains stable or decreases with increasing age during adulthood. As age increases past 60, consumption levels are lower and alcohol abuse is less prevalent. Some reasons proposed for decreases in consumption by older persons include chronic health problems, decreased income, increased sensitivity to the effects of alcohol, lifestyle changes associated with retirement, and the influence of peers' drinking patterns (USDHHS, 1990).

ALCOHOL USE AMONG ATHLETES

Although frequently a topic in the popular media, alcohol use among athletes is not often critically examined. The following subsections discuss alcohol use among athletes at the secondary, collegiate or amateur, and professional levels and compare their use with the general population.

Secondary Level

Is there reason for concern over the level of alcohol use by middle and high school athletes relative to their peers? Although few investigations have focused on this issue, recent studies suggest that there are reasons for concern over alcohol use by secondary school athletes. Carr, Kennedy, and Dimick (1990), reporting results of a survey of senior high school students, found that male athletes consumed alcohol significantly more than male nonathletes. There was no difference found in alcohol use by female athletes and nonathletes. There also was no difference found in the reported experience of intoxication between athletes and nonathletes; however, male athletes reported intoxication significantly more than female athletes. Similarly, Ringwalt (1988) in a survey of high school students in North Carolina found that athletes were more likely to use alcohol and to be intoxicated in the 30 days before the survey, even though rate of lifetime use and of intoxication for athletes and nonathletes was the same. Also of concern was that both athletes and nonathletes gave the lowest risk ratings to alcohol use compared with other drug use, suggesting that they perceived alcohol use as a relatively risk free activity.

In a more recent study of North Carolina high school youth, Mikow and Raven (1993) found no significant differences between athletes and nonathletes in their lifetime use of alcohol and other drugs. However, male athletes were significantly more likely to use alcohol of any type, as well as smokeless tobacco, marijuana, and steroids, than female athletes. These investigators also found that one-fourth of athletes and nonathletes reported having tried beer and cigarettes before the 7th grade. Furthermore, when comparing their results with the Ringwalt (1988) results, they found that a significantly greater percentage of 11th- and 12th-grade athletes in 1991, relative to 1988, reported experimentation (lifetime use) with cigarettes and alcohol of any type.

These survey results suggest that high school athletes are using alcohol at least at a rate comparable to their peers and that male athletes may be using alcohol more frequently than their male, nonathlete counterparts. Also, male athletes appear to be drinking to intoxication at a rate comparable to their male peers and significantly more than female athletes. Therefore, male athletes appear to be a subpopulation of youth with particular risks for alcohol-related problems. There is also indication that experimentation with alcohol and cigarettes is occurring before entry into secondary school by both athletes and nonathletes. Alcohol use appears to be related to use of other drugs (smokeless tobacco, marijuana, steroids) in male athletes.

Collegiate and Amateur Level

Just as with secondary school level athletes, alcohol use by collegiate and amateur athletes appears at least at a level of their nonathlete peers. Anderson, Albrecht, McKeag, Hough, and McGrew (1991) surveyed college athletes at 11 institutions in five men's and five women's sports and found that 89 percent of athletes reported alcohol use in the preceding 12 months. A similar survey conducted in the mid-1980s by Anderson and McKeag (as cited in Anderson et al., 1991) found 88 percent of student and amateur athletes reporting alcohol use in the preceding 12 months, suggesting alcohol use had remained fairly stable in this population. Anderson et al. also found that alcohol was by far the most used drug among college athletes when compared with cocaine, crack, marijuana, hashish, smokeless tobacco, amphetamines, anabolic steroids, major pain medications (e.g., Tylenol #3, Percodan, morphine, etc.), and prescription weight loss products (e.g., Dexatrim, Acutrim, etc.). Unfortunately, the survey did not ask the participants about caffeine and nicotine (in cigarettes). The researchers found that alcohol use during the previous 12 months among athletes was somewhat lower but comparable to alcohol use reported by college students in a national survey conducted by Johnston, O'Malley, and Bachman (as cited in Anderson et al., 1991). Table 2.2 demonstrates this comparison for alcohol and other drugs and indicates the vast difference between reported alcohol and other drug use. Ninety percent of male athletes reported alcohol use in the preceding 12 months compared to 93 percent of male college students. Eighty-seven percent of female athletes reported use during the preceding year compared to 90 percent of female college students. Athletes reported less use of cocaine, crack, marijuana, and hashish than their nonathlete peers. Anderson et al. (1991) indicated that there was a significant decrease in the reported use of these drugs by athletes from 1985 to 1989. The authors suggested that decreased cocaine and crack use by athletes may have been partly attributable to increased awareness of the dangers associated with this drug's use. In the case of marijuana and hashish, the authors speculated that decreased use may have been because of drug-testing efforts or a simultaneous drop in use by the general population.

Other studies of athlete and nonathlete drinking among college students lend support to the idea that alcohol use by athletes and nonathletes is similar. For instance, Overman and Terry (1991) found no significant differences in alcohol use between athletes and nonathletes in a study of students from two state universities and two private colleges. However, these investigators found evidence suggesting that drinking patterns may vary between athletes and nonathletes. For instance, they found that male nonathletes drank significantly more during the week than male athletes, who tended to drink more on weekends and special occasions. In addition, they found that athletes reported drinking more beer than nonathletes, perhaps, as the authors suggested, reflecting influences of marketing strategies of beer distributors or traditional values associated with participation in sport. They also found that drinking patterns of

TABLE 2.2

Drug Use by Varsity Athletes at 11 NCAA Schools During Previous
12 Months Compared With Drug Use by General Population
of College Students

	VARSITY ATHLETES		COLLEGE STUDENTS	
Drugs	Males, % (n = 1552)	Females, % (n = 730)	Males, % (n = 520)	Females, % (n = 700)
Alcohol	90	87	93	90
Amphetamines	3	3	7	7
Cocaine or crack	6	4	19	14
Marijuana or hashish	29	25	41	34

Note. From "A National Survey of Alcohol and Drug Use by College Athletes" by W. A. Anderson, R. R. Albrecht, D. B. McKeag, D. O. Hough, and C. A. McGrew, 1991, *Physician and Sportsmedicine,* 19(2), p. 101. Copyright 1991 by McGraw Hill Healthcare. Adapted by permission.

subgroups of nonathletes differed more than subgroups of athletes. The authors suggested that participation in athletics may have the effect of socializing all athletes toward similar drinking behaviors. The study showed this by the fact that male and female athletes' alcohol use appeared to be more similar than male and female nonathletes. Finally, this study found that college athletes' attitudes toward alcohol did not correlate with their drinking behavior. Despite athletes believing that drinking was harmful to health, relative to nonathletes, they did not drink less than nonathletes.

Although data regarding amateur, noncollegiate athletes use of alcohol is less available, there are reports suggesting that alcohol use is common among some amateur athletes and frequently may exceed average population consumption levels. A survey of subscribers to *Runner's World* (Stewart, 1981) found that 40 percent of respondents reported drinking a six-pack of beer or less a week, 20 percent drank one to three six-packs a week, and 4 percent drank more than that a week. Thirty-three percent reported not drinking beer at all. A study conducted at Stanford University's Heart Disease Prevention Program cited by Stewart (1981) suggested that runners drank twice as much beer as non-runners, which meant they averaged about four glasses of beer daily. Unfortunately, both studies were cited in a trade publication, *Runner's World*, which means that methodological description was unavailable and therefore interpretation of results is difficult. Rugby players have been heavy consumers of beer before and after a match (Thomson, 1977). Survey data have suggested that drinkers are overrepresented among rugby players. Indeed, Frey (1973) found that 100 percent of amateur, noncollegiate rugby players responded affirmatively to the question, "Do you drink alcoholic beverages?"

Professional Level

Although reports of alcohol and other drug abuse among professional athletes are common in the media, few studies have been done to clarify the rates of alcohol use in this population. In a survey of 262 male members of a professional sport league (which league was not reported by the author) regarding their use of alcohol and other drugs, including nicotine in cigarettes, nighttime cold medicines, marijuana, hashish, and cocaine, Malone (1991) found that alcohol was the only drug that many players reported using regularly. Except for alcohol, Malone found a sharp decrease in reported drug use from lifetime use, to 12-month use, to use within the past 30 days. Virtually all the respondents (99.6 percent) reported lifetime use of alcohol, and 93 percent reported alcohol use in the last 30 days. Approximately one-third of the athletes reported two or more drinking occasions in the last two weeks when they consumed five or more drinks in a row. Also, those athletes reporting alcohol use within the last 30 days tended to consume alcohol frequently. The author indicated that comparing this group of players with a similar age group in the general population suggested that a greater percentage of the athletes reported using alcohol. However, the reported use of other drugs in the last 12 months by athletes was much lower than their age mates in the general population.

The results of Malone's (1991) study indicate that alcohol was clearly the drug of choice among the male professional athletes surveyed. In addition, 40 (15 percent) of the respondents of the survey were rated as problem drinkers based on their responses to the Michigan Alcoholism Screening Test, a frequently used self-report instrument designed to screen for problem drinking. A participant observer study conducted by Gallmeier (1988) further suggests that heavy alcohol use is not uncommon among professional athletes. Gallmeier spent the 1981–1982 hockey season conducting his study with a group of minor league hockey players. Essentially, the author became part of the hockey team during the season, participating in "all the activities that the players were involved in with the exception of actually playing the game" (Gallmeier, 1988, p. 2). During the study, he met 75 players ranging in age from 19 to 30. He found that the most common drug activity among the players involved team drinking sessions following all home games and most road games. "The players called these events 'juicing sessions' and believed they were necessary for developing team solidarity" (Gallmeier, 1988, p. 3). These studies, one based on survey data and the other on behavioral observation, along with reports in the news media (Byrd, 1991a, 1991b), suggest that alcohol is a frequently used drug by professional athletes and that it may pose a significant problem for some athletes.

Attitudes Toward and Reasons for Alcohol Use

There are three primary reasons athletes use drugs: (a) as ergogenic aids to facilitate physical performance, (b) as restorative agents to allow continued performance despite injury, and (c) as recreational drugs to cope with problems or to experience altered mental or physical states (Nuzzo & Waller, 1988). Though it is difficult to place alcohol solely in one of the three categories, its use by athletes is generally for recreational purposes. However, in some instances athletes may use alcohol for performance-enhancing reasons (e.g., by pistol shooters as a means of decreasing anxiety and steadying hand tremors). Chapter 3 will specifically address performance effects of alcohol.

Although previous research (e.g., Hayes & Tevis, 1977) found that nonathletes held more tolerant attitudes toward alcohol use and reported greater incidence of heavy drinking than athletes, more recent findings (Rooney, 1984; Stuck, 1988) have suggested that nonathletes and athletes are more similar than dissimilar in their attitudes toward and use of alcohol. Indeed, it has been suggested that sport is a microcosm of the social world and reflects the profile of American life existing at the time (Edwards, 1973). Therefore, when drug and alcohol use are part of the social fabric, we can expect them to be part of the sport world as well.

Similar to the general population, reasons for alcohol use by athletes differ depending on age and circumstances. In a recent study of high school athletes (Green, Burke, Nix, Lambrecht, and Mason, 1995), some reasons reported for alcohol use were to have a good time with friends, to celebrate, to feel good, and to deal with the pressures of school and athletics. Although not reported as a reason for drinking by high school athletes, alcohol use may help the athlete cope with anxiety-provoking social situations. Hover and Gaffney (1991) found that adolescent drinkers differed from nondrinkers in their level of social skills, with drinkers having lower social skills than nondrinkers and problem drinkers having the lowest level of social skills. Their study did not determine whether low-level social skills were a cause or consequence of drinking; however, the results suggest that for some drinkers alcohol may serve a role in helping them to compensate for a deficit in social skills. The inclusion of social skills training in many alcohol rehabilitation programs supports the notion that lack of social skills may prompt alcohol use or abuse (Monti, Gulliver, & Myers, 1994).

Not surprisingly, collegiate athletes report similar reasons to high school athletes for using alcohol. In a survey of collegiate athletes' drug use, Evans, Weinberg, and Jackson (1992) found that respondents cited three primary reasons for alcohol use. Seventy-eight percent said they used alcohol for recreation and social reasons, 47 percent indicated they used alcohol to feel good, and 28 percent said they used alcohol to deal with stress from college life. This study also found that those athletes who used alcohol the most scored significantly higher on the subscales of anger, fatigue, and vigor on the Profile of Mood States (POMS), a questionnaire designed to measure six major mood states. Although the authors did not regard the differences between high-alcohol and low-alcohol users on the vigor subscale as a significant factor in athlete alcohol use, the differences between the two groups on anger and fatigue were noteworthy. These findings suggest that alcohol use by collegiate athletes may in part be an effort to deal with negative mental and physical states such as anger and fatigue. In addition, Evans et al. (1992) found that male high-alcohol-using athletes reported feeling significantly more pressure to perform well from coaches than low-user or nonuser male athletes, who reported more pressure from maintaining grades necessary to remain eligible. Given this perceived pressure to perform athletically in high-alcohol-using male athletes, it is reasonable to assume that some athletes may use alcohol to relieve this pressure (Roberts-Wilbur, Wilbur, & Morris as cited in Evans et al., 1992).

Reasons for alcohol use among professional athletes are not unlike their junior colleagues, but their reasons tend to be more variable. Malone (1991) found that athletes in a professional sport league that she surveyed reported using alcohol and drugs (in order of most frequently reported) to relax or relieve tensions, to have a good time with friends, to experiment, to feel good or get high, and to fit in with the group. She also asked these athletes to report on their reasons for not using or stopping use of drugs and alcohol. Their top five reasons were no need for it, against their beliefs, concerned about health, don't like it, and illegal. Another reason given for stopping alcohol use only was recognizing it was becoming a problem.

In his study of professional hockey players, Gallmeier (1988) found that reasons for alcohol use were dealing with idle time, developing team solidarity, and promoting free expression of feelings. A quote from one of the players best exemplifies these apparent reasons for alcohol use:

> *A lot of guys drink heavily because there is so much free time. You know we practice in the morning for maybe an hour then we go out to lunch and have one beer, then another one, and then it just goes on eh? You see it's very important to be together as a team. I've played on teams where you spend the whole year not getting to know each other. But if you are on a team which goes out and parties together it's better. Bars are places where you can do that as a team eh? You let loose your feelings. I think it's good. Close knit relationships all happen in a bar. That's how you get to know each other. (Gallmeier, 1988, p. 3–4)*

ALCOHOL USE AMONG SPORT PROFESSIONALS

Although it is not the central focus of this book, when discussing the alcohol use habits of athletes, it is also important to consider the patterns of alcohol use by sport professionals, who are often significant to the athlete. These professionals include coaches, sport administrators, and health professionals involved in treating injured athletes or athletes with alcohol-related or other mental health problems. How these individuals use alcohol may serve as a model for athletes and may influence whether these professionals can accurately identify problematic drinking patterns in athletes and intervene appropriately (cf. Romney & Bynner, 1985).

There is a lack of documentation of alcohol use by coaches and sport administrators. Therefore, one is left to assume that their alcohol use approximates the general population. We can support a similar estimation for health professionals with some exceptions. For example, in a recent review of studies of substance use and addiction among medical students, residents, and physicians, Flaherty and Richman (1993) found that alcohol-related problems increased with age among physicians as opposed to the general population, which shows a decrease of alcohol-related problems over time. Also of note and concern is the apparent lack of gender differences in problematic drinking among medical students, with the pattern of drinking rates for women approximating that for men by the end of medical school.

A recent study of physician drinking habits (McAuliffe et al., 1991) not cited by Flaherty and Richman (1993) found that older male doctors qualified more frequently as heavy drinkers than younger male doctors (a finding inconsistent with the general population) and found that males drank more than females (a finding consistent with the general population). The results of these recent studies do not suggest significant differences in overall alcohol use and abuse between physicians and the general population. However, it appears that, unlike the general population in which alcohol consumption decreases with age, alcohol consumption for male physicians increases with age. Also, there is some evidence that women in medical training respond to this experience with increased problematic drinking. Although on one level it may be encouraging news that physicians do not use alcohol more than the general population, given the critical nature of their activities, alcohol use rates at the general population level may present problems in the discharge of their responsibilities. Increased alcohol use by older male doctors is of particular concern because their responsibilities and influence are likely to increase with age.

ALCOHOL USE AMONG SPORT SPECTATORS

Spectators are an integral part of the sport experience in the United States, particularly in Division I National Collegiate Athletic Association (NCAA) and professional levels. Though spectators are not directly part of the competition, their financial support of athletics and their behavior during sport events have significant influence on the conditions under which athletes compete.

Alcohol consumption by spectators at sport events is commonplace, even if sale and possession of alcohol inside the stadium or arena is prohibited. Starting with tailgate parties in the parking lot and ending with after-game celebrations or commiserations, alcohol is an accustomed ingredient in the sport experience for many spectators.

In recent years there has been growing concern expressed in the media and by collegiate administrators and professional league officials about the effects of spectator drinking on sport events. Johnson (1993) chronicled the *celebrations* following the championships of the Chicago Bulls, Montreal Canadiens, and the Dallas Cowboys in 1993 and described the tragedies associated with fans out of control. Similar instances of soccer fans rioting after major competitions have caused concern among sport and police officials (Ward, 1990). Rugby officials also have expressed concern that rugby fans may be emulating their counterparts in soccer (Parry-Jones, 1980).

Without exception, alcohol use has been a common factor associated with these episodes of fan violence directed toward themselves, players, and property. Though most fans consuming alcoholic beverages while attending sport events do not cause harm to their environment, the incidence of violence has been sufficient to warrant actions to prevent or contain alcohol-related incidents. Perhaps stimulated by potential legal liability, as exemplified by relevant court cases ("New Jersey," 1987; Wong & Ensor, 1985), sport administrators have begun to take action to reduce the likelihood of alcohol-related problems at sport events. For instance, Major League Baseball, the National Basketball Association, the National Football League, the National Hockey League, the National Collegiate Athletic Association (NCAA), and a variety of private, public, and volunteer agencies are members of Techniques for Effective Alcohol Management (TEAM), an organization dedicated to reducing alcohol misuse in and around public facilities ("Alcohol-Related Incidents," 1991). Although we cannot expect that alcohol-related incidents will be eliminated entirely, these are important steps by institutions to curb the potential problems that alcohol use may cause for those involved in planning and participating in sport events. Chapter 5 will discuss these and other preventive measures in greater detail.

CONCLUSION

A strong relationship has developed over the years between alcohol and sport, prompted in part by a beneficial relationship between sport organizations and beer breweries. Most data suggest that alcohol use among sport-related populations approximates use in the general population. However, because alcohol use among the general population causes significant negative consequences, it may be that as a society we should reduce alcohol consumption within the sport context, particularly because many athletes occupy influential positions within our social structure.

In chapter 3, we will explore the biomedical and behavioral effects of alcohol, its effects on human performance, and specifically its influence on sport performance. This chapter will provide additional information about whether athletes and others involved in sport should more closely evaluate their use of alcohol.

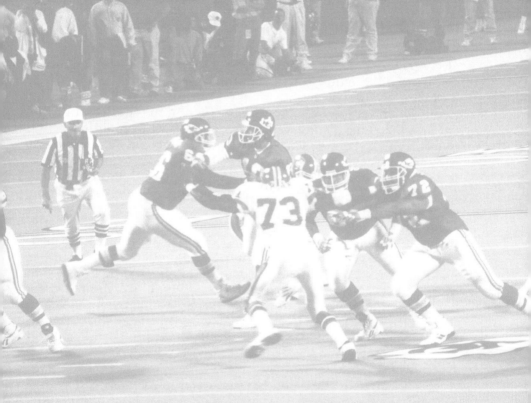

3 ALCOHOL, HUMAN FUNCTIONING, AND SPORT PERFORMANCE

I can drink without danger, I am so near to the ground.

—Henri Toulouse-Lautrec

In chapter 2, we explored the various aspects that have linked alcohol to sport in the United States and reviewed alcohol use in sport populations. In this chapter, we will examine alcohol's influence on the human body, on behavior, on human performance generally, and on sport performance specifically. This chapter is purposely broad so the reader will understand the impact of alcohol on human functioning. This understanding will provide the context from which to extrapolate to the effects of alcohol on sport performance.

BIOMEDICAL EFFECTS OF ALCOHOL

Although it is beyond the scope of this chapter to comprehensively cover the biomedical effects of alcohol, the following overview will include how alcohol is absorbed and metabolized, its primary sites of action, major pharmacological effects, the development of tolerance to its effects, characteristics of physical and psychological dependence, and how alcohol affects primary organ systems. The interested reader can find excellent reviews of these topics in Blum (1984), Corry and Cimbolic (1985), Mannaioni (1984), and Ray and Ksir (1993). Williams (1994) and "Lesser"(1993) contain reviews specific to the influence of alcohol on organ systems.

Alcohol is absorbed unaltered, rapidly, and directly into the body, starting with small amounts of absorption in the mouth. Most alcohol is absorbed through the stomach and the upper small intestine. The rate of absorption is affected by the type of alcoholic beverage and the speed with which it is consumed; the concentration of alcohol in the beverage; stomach contents and factors that influence stomach emptying time (e.g., carbonation of the beverage, nausea, condition of the stomach tissue, and emotional states such as fear and anger); body weight; and gastric motility.

Alcohol crosses the blood-brain barrier immediately, depressing the central nervous system (CNS) almost instantaneously. Alcohol is distributed quickly and unchanged throughout the body fluids, tissues, and organs. Therefore, heavier people will experience less psychoactive effects of alcohol because body mass reduces the concentration of alcohol in the bloodstream. Over 90 percent of alcohol ingested is eliminated from the body through metabolism in the liver. A small amount of alcohol (less than 10 percent) is excreted unchanged in the urine, sweat, and breath.

Unlike most other drugs, metabolism of alcohol occurs at a constant rate regardless of the concentration of alcohol in the blood (blood alcohol concentration, or BAC, also referred to as blood alcohol level, or BAL). This metabolic rate for an adult is approximately .25 to .3 oz (7 to 10 g) of 100 percent alcohol per hour. Although the metabolic rate of alcohol is constant in the individual, there are individual differences in response to alcohol (and other drugs) because of variations in liver enzyme systems responsible for metabolism, which are affected by age, menstrual cycle, race, heredity, liver disease, and experience with alcohol and other drug consumption. The rate of metabolism is important in determining the time required to function without behavioral decrements. Specific BAC ranges are associated with common behavioral decrements, which we will discuss in a later section on behavioral effects of alcohol.

Pharmacology of Alcohol

The acute pharmacological effects of alcohol are numerous, with many having direct potential bearing on sport performance. For example, alcohol dilates blood vessels close to the skin surface, therefore increasing heat loss in cold weather. Also, if consumed in sufficient quantities, alcohol directly suppresses the body's temperature regulatory mechanism. Because of these effects it is not advisable to use alcohol to stay warm in a cold climate.

At high BAC, alcohol may reduce the heart's ability to contract. Alcohol also changes blood lipoproteins, which may explain the apparent reduced risk of heart attack in moderate drinkers compared with abstainers or heavy drinkers. Although this finding suggests moderate alcohol use may have some health benefits regarding prevention of heart disease, other adverse health effects of alcohol, as well as the possibility of abuse, preclude a recommendation to increase alcohol use or begin drinking if one currently abstains (see review by Williams, 1994).

Alcohol has an anticoagulant effect, therefore increasing blood loss rate in the event of injury. The diuretic effect of alcohol leads to increases in volume of urine produced when BAC increases. This effect of alcohol may disturb electrolyte balance and lead to dehydration. Alcohol also raises the seizure threshold level while BAC is increasing. However, as BAC decreases, threshold levels are reduced, which may prompt withdrawal seizures in a recently abstinent heavy drinker. Alcohol suppresses rapid eye movement (REM) sleep. Disturbed sleep may occur when drinking stops, which relates to the phenomenon of REM rebound (a period when REM sleep temporarily increases above normal levels in response to recent REM sleep deprivation). Alcohol interacts with numerous drugs and is most dangerous when combined with other CNS depressants, leading to a potentiating effect that may arrest breathing.

As drinking increases in frequency and volume, tolerance for many effects of alcohol will occur. Tolerance refers to the phenomenon of the drinker requiring increasing doses of alcohol over time to produce the same effects lesser doses produced previously. Tolerance is believed to develop through metabolic, cellular, and behavioral processes. The metabolic process refers to increased activity in liver enzymes responsible for metabolizing alcohol, which causes the liver to oxidize alcohol more efficiently. At the cellular level, a process of accommodation to the effects of alcohol occurs, enabling the cells to function despite the presence of alcohol. Behavioral tolerance or *holding your liquor* refers to the individual's ability to function despite high BAC. It has been conjectured that alcoholism may be a specific tolerance abnormality that prevents the individual from drinking in a normal fashion (Tabakoff & Hoffman, 1988).

As tolerance develops, risk for psychological or physical dependence on alcohol increases. Both types of dependence occur on a continuum of severity. Psychological dependence refers to the individual's perceived need for alcohol as a coping tool. This perceived need typically will increase over time as drinking frequency and volume increase. Physical dependence is characterized by withdrawal symptoms when drinking stops. When a hangover occurs after a bout of drinking, one is experiencing a mild form of withdrawal from alcohol. In the average drinker this syndrome will run its course in a day and the individual will return to normal functioning. The chronic heavy drinker, however, often treats a hangover with the most available and effective remedy—alcohol. As this self-medication of hangover continues, the severity of physical dependence increases. When the chronic heavy drinker stops drinking, withdrawal from alcohol occurs, characterized by autonomic nervous system arousal (e.g., increased heart rate and blood pressure, profuse sweating, tremors), and, in severe cases, visual, auditory and tactile hallucinations, delusions, disorientation, and seizures. Depending on the history of the individual, treatment of withdrawal may require hospitalization.

Alcohol's Effects on Organ Systems, Fetal Development, and Cancer Risk

This section will provide an overview of the effects of alcohol on primary organ systems, fetal development, and cancer risk. This topic has received extensive attention in the medical literature, so do not regard the following as complete coverage of this literature. The beginning of this section noted general references for more information on these topics.

Central Nervous System. Alcohol has acute and chronic effects on the CNS. It is a CNS depressant, leading to sedation in lower doses and sleep and coma in higher doses. Higher centers of the brain are depressed initially, affecting speech, thought, restraint, and judgment. Lower brain centers are affected as BAC rises, slowing respiration and reflexes. The effects of chronic heavy alcohol use on the CNS may be devastating. These effects include disorganization of neuronal membrane structure, which alters conduction rates of nerve impulses; peripheral neuropathy, which results in pain and sensory complaints; cortical atrophy (reduction in the size of the cortex), which has been found in alcoholic inpatients on autopsy; sleep disturbance caused by the effects of alcohol on REM sleep; and CNS disorders such as Wernicke-Korsakoff syndrome, which is characterized by various neurological symptoms and severe memory loss. This syndrome is associated with deficiency of the vitamin B thiamine brought on by poor nutrition common in alcoholics.

Cardiovascular System. Alcohol also may adversely affect the cardiovascular system. Hypertension has been associated with heavy drinking as well as a form of cardiomyopathy (damage to the heart muscle) caused by chronic heavy drinking or related nutritional deficiencies. Alcohol in intoxicating doses also has been associated with cardiac arrhythmias, which may cause sudden heart failure in individuals with or without a history of heart disease (Friedman, 1992). Alcohol in moderate doses (which is defined differently across studies) has been suggested as a protective agent for cardiovascular risk; however, the complications of alcohol use may outweigh these potential positive effects.

Gastrointestinal System. Alcohol affects the gastrointestinal system in a variety of ways. At low concentrations, alcohol stimulates the gastric lining to produce acid that may aid digestion. At higher concentrations, the secretion of mucus is increased, stomach mucosa becomes congested, and acid production decreases, which may result in acute gastritis. Prolonged heavy alcohol use may yield nutritional complications because of interference with nutrient absorption. The pancreas is directly affected by heavy alcohol use, which may lead to hypoglycemia and severe pancreatic damage often found in alcoholics.

Because of its major role in the metabolism of alcohol, the liver is often the site of extensive damage in the chronic heavy drinker. Conditions such as alcoholic hepatitis, fatty liver, and cirrhosis are often the result of chronic, long-term heavy drinking. Although mortality from chronic liver disease and cirrhosis has been declining during the last 20 years in the United States and many other developed countries, in 1988 cirrhosis was the ninth leading cause of death in the United States (Grant, DeBakey, & Zobeck, 1991).

Reproductive System. The reproductive system in men is affected by alcohol, leading to testosterone suppression and to testicular atrophy in some heavy drinkers. In women who drink heavily there are frequent gynecological complaints. In general, chronic heavy drinking interferes with sexual desire and response. It is not uncommon for those in treatment for alcohol dependence or abuse to report significant problems in their sexual functioning and relationships with partners. Excellent reviews of the effects of heavy alcohol use on male and female sexual functioning are contained in Schiavi (1990) and Roman (1988a), respectively.

Immune System. Finally, alcohol has inhibitory effects on the immune system, which may in part account for alcoholics' increased risk for infection. This effect of alcohol on the immune system, combined with other potential negative physical effects of alcohol and its influence on risk-taking behavior, increase an individual's risk of disease. A recent issue of *Alcohol, Health & Research World* ("Alcohol," 1992) reviews research that links alcohol use with increased risk for contracting the human immunodeficiency virus (HIV) infection and the onset of acquired immune deficiency syndrome (AIDS), bacterial pneumonia, cancer, tuberculosis, and viral hepatitis. Although the relationship between alcohol consumption, changes in the immune system, and infection have not been clearly delineated, it appears that alcohol use, particularly in higher volumes, is a risk factor for a compromised immune system.

Alcohol and Fetal Malformation. Negative effects of alcohol on fetal development have been documented in the last 20 years. We can group associated abnormalities into four categories: CNS dysfunction, birth deficiencies, facial abnormalities, and various major and minor malformations (Goodwin, 1992). Although the role of alcohol in the etiology of the so-called fetal alcohol syndrome remains controversial, most clinicians would likely caution women against excessive drinking during pregnancy and perhaps would counsel abstinence, because safe levels of alcohol have not been determined.

Alcohol and Cancer. The literature notes increases in risk for cancer in heavy drinkers (see review in NIAAA, 1993). Alcohol has been linked to cancer, particularly cancers of the upper digestive tract, including the mouth, esophagus, pharynx, and larynx. Less consistent relationships have been found linking alcohol consumption to cancers of the liver, breast, and colon. Cancer risk is magnified for people who smoke and drink. For example, risk for mouth, tracheal, and esophageal cancer is 35 times greater for people who smoke and drink (two or more packs of cigarettes and more than four alcoholic drinks per day) than for people who do neither (Blot et al., 1988).

With these potential negative physical effects of alcohol, a question may come to mind whether there is a safe amount of alcohol one can consume without suffering ill effects. This subject has been debated for many years, and presently we have no definite answers regarding safe amounts. Because we don't fully understand the risk factors for developing alcohol dependence, it is safest either to abstain from alcohol consumption or confine one's drinking to specific, circumscribed occasions, preferably with food consumption.

BEHAVIORAL EFFECTS OF ALCOHOL

Because alcohol is absorbed directly into the bloodstream, primarily through the stomach and small intestine, and is distributed throughout the body, its effects on behavior are immediate. Individual differences in response to the effects of alcohol are primarily based on gender (women are typically more suscepti-ble to the effects of alcohol) and metabolic tolerance to alcohol.

The sites of action of alcohol within the CNS are widespread and nonspecific. Alcohol essentially depresses all brain cells. In low doses it depresses inhibitory centers in the brain, thereby producing subjective feelings of confidence and perhaps eupho-ria. However, there is much individual variation in these effects of alcohol. Following initial depression of inhibitory centers, excitatory brain centers are suppressed, yielding behavioral depressant effects such as sleepiness and impaired motor coor-dination (Corry & Cimbolic, 1985). The effects of alcohol on exci-tatory centers are dose dependent (i.e., the more alcohol ingest-ed, the greater the excitatory depression).

As noted earlier in this chapter, BAC is the measurement used to determine the concentration of alcohol in the blood-stream. Levels of BAC are expressed as the number of grams (g) of alcohol per 100 milliliters (ml) of blood and are usually indi-cated as a percentage. Therefore, since 100 g in 100 ml would equal 100 percent, 100 milligrams (mg) of alcohol in 100 ml of blood would be reported as 0.10 percent or 100 mg percent (Ray & Ksir, 1993). In most states, a BAC at the .10 level is inter-preted as legally intoxicated. BAC is estimated by samples of blood, urine, breath, or saliva. For purposes of this book, we will express levels of BAC in numeric form only (e.g., .10 represents 100 mg/100 ml or 100 mg percent).

Variables such as sex, weight, and period in the menstrual cycle may affect BAC. Table 3.1 indicates approximate levels of BAC that we might expect as a result of sex, body weight, and number and type of alcoholic beverages consumed, assuming there is no tolerance to alcohol. This table assumes standard drink quantities of .5 oz of pure alcohol (see chapter 1, p. 3 for beverage equivalents).

Various levels of BAC are associated with different behavioral effects (see table 3.2). As the table suggests, the initial effects of alcohol are typically relaxation and mild euphoria, and as BAC increases, there are progressively greater decrements in behav-ioral measures. At the higher levels of BAC (.30–.45), the indi-vidual loses consciousness and may die from respiratory failure at levels approximating .45.

In addition to alcohol's effects on behavior noted in table 3.2, one's expectancy (expectation) regarding alcohol's effects also plays a major role in how alcohol influences behavior. Marlatt (1987) reviewed the literature on the effects of expectancies

TABLE 3.1

Relationships Among Gender, Weight, Alcohol Consumption, and Blood Alcohol Level							
		BLOOD ALCOHOL LEVELS (G/100 ML)					
Absolute alcohol (oz)	Beverage Intake per hour	Female (100 lb)	Male (100 lb)	Female (150 lb)	Male (150 lb)	Female (200 lb)	Male (200 lb)
1/2	1 oz spirits‡ 1 glass wine 1 can beer	0.045	0.037	0.03	0.025	0.022	0.019
1	2 oz spirits 2 glasses wine 2 cans beer	0.090	0.075	0.06	0.050	0.045	0.037
2	4 oz spirits 4 glasses wine 4 cans beer	0.180	0.150	0.12	0.100	0.090	0.070
3	6 oz spirits 6 glasses wine 6 cans beer	0.270	0.220	0.18	0.150	0.130	0.110
4	8 oz spirits 8 glasses wine 8 cans beer	0.360	0.300	0.24	0.200	0.180	0.150
5	10 oz spirits 10 glasses wine 10 cans beer	0.450	0.370	0.30	0.250	0.220	0.180

‡100-proof spirits.

From *Drugs, Society, & Human Behavior* (p. 194) by O. Ray and C. Ksir, 1993, St. Louis, MO: Mosby-Year Book. Copyright 1993 by Mosby-Year Book. Reprinted with permission.

about alcohol and found them to powerfully influence emotional and behavioral states while drinking. This research area continues to receive considerable attention and may help to delineate the role that expectancies play in developing alcohol abuse and alcohol dependence and in recovering from these problems.

Acute Effects

Prominent, acute cognitive and behavioral effects of alcohol are on memory, coordination, social behavior, and tendency toward aggression. With regard to memory, the acute effects typically

TABLE 3.2

Blood Alcohol Level and Behavioral Effects	
Present blood alcohol level	**Average effects**
.02	Reached after approximately one drink; light or moderate drinkers experience some pleasant feelings (e.g., sense of warmth and well-being).
.04	Most people feel relaxed, energetic, and happy. Time seems to pass quickly. Skin may flush, and motor skills may be slightly impaired.
.05	More observable effects begin to occur. Individual may experience lightheartedness, giddiness, lowered inhibitions, and impaired judgment. Coordination may be slightly altered.
.06	Further impairment of judgment; individual's ability to make rational decisions concerning personal capabilities is affected (e.g., driving a car). May become "a lover or a fighter."
.08	Muscle coordination definitely impaired and reaction time increased; driving ability suspect. Heavy pulse and slow breathing. Sensory feelings of numbness in the cheeks, lips, and extremities may occur.
.10	Clear deterioration of coordination and reaction time. Individual may stagger and speech may become fuzzy. Judgment and memory further affected (legally *drunk*, in most states).
.15	All individuals experience a definite impairment of balance and movement. Large increases in reaction time.
.20	Marked depression in motor and sensory capability; slurred speech, double vision, difficulty standing and walking may all be present. Decidedly intoxicated.
.30	Individual is confused or stuperous; unable to comprehend what is seen or heard. May lose consciousness (passes out) at this level.
.40	Usually unconscious. Alcohol has become deep anesthetic. Skin may be sweaty and clammy.
.45	Circulatory and respiration functions are depressed and can stop altogether.
.50	Near death.

From *Drugs: Facts, Alternatives, Decisions* (p. 171) by J.M. Corry and P. Cimbolic, 1985, Belmont, CA: Wadsworth Publishing Company. Copyright 1985 by Wadsworth Publishing Company. Reprinted with permission.

impair encoding and retrieval processes. Therefore, experiences are not well encoded in the brain, and the ability to retrieve what is encoded is impaired. Alcohol's effect on social and aggressive behavior has been described as biphasic. That is, at lower levels of BAC, it is common for the individual to become more jovial and gregarious and possibly to take uncharacteristic risks in a social setting. Increased drinking, however, leads to increased disinhibition resulting from suppressed higher centers of the cortex responsible for inhibiting behavior. The result is greater probability of aggressive behavior. These effects of alcohol on social and aggressive behavior, combined with alcohol-related deficiencies in coordination, may be responsible for the decrements in motor performance that often result in motor vehicle accidents. For example, despite reaching a 17-year (1977–1993) low, 35.5 percent of traffic crash deaths in 1993 were alcohol related. During that period, the mean BAC for drivers involved in fatal crashes was .16 (Campbell, Zobeck, & Bertolucci, 1995). It is important to remember that all these acute effects of alcohol occur in individuals with or without alcoholism and in most cases are reversible with abstinence.

Effects of Chronic Heavy Drinking

The effects of chronic alcoholism on cognitive and behavioral functioning are variable. Recent neuropsychological literature supports the existence of three categories of organic brain disease associated with prolonged alcoholism: Wernicke-Korsakoff syndrome, alcoholic dementia, and *nonamnesic* or *non-Korsakoff* disorders (USDHHS, 1993). These categories are distinguished by the presence or absence of amnesia and the extent of associated intellectual impairment. Wernicke-Korsakoff syndrome is typified by severe memory impairment with relatively intact intellectual functioning; alcoholic dementia involves global intellectual decline along with severe memory deficits. The third grouping of chronic alcoholics has been referred to as neurologically asymptomatic (Bowden, 1990) and is characterized by a lack of obvious signs of severe cognitive impairment. Alcoholics in this group may show deficits in abstract reasoning, problem solving, visuoperceptual skills, and mild learning and memory impairments (Parsons, Butters, & Nathan, 1987).

These disorders associated with alcoholism most likely relate to neurotoxic effects of alcohol or vitamin deficiencies from malnutrition (particularly thiamine) or both. Factors contributing to individual susceptibility to alcohol-related brain damage as well as the underlying cerebral mechanisms responsible for the observed deficits are yet to be fully elucidated (USDHHS, 1993). Significant recovery from these disorders may occur with continued abstinence.

Effects of Social Drinking

The literature has paid recent attention to the potential negative consequences on cognitive functioning of social drinking (averaging one or two drinks per day or more). In a review of this literature, Parsons (1986) indicated that there is no consistent evidence to support the idea that social drinking causes altered cognitive functioning when drinkers are sober. Even though this review is a decade old, its conclusion still appears valid. However, as Parsons stresses, this does not mean that we should stop investigating the hypothesized relationship between social drinking and altered cognitive functioning. Social drinking is far too commonplace to ignore its possible negative or positive consequences on cognitive functioning and general health.

EFFECTS OF ALCOHOL ON HUMAN PERFORMANCE

As we might expect based on the previous discussion of physical and behavioral effects of alcohol, human performance in a variety of tasks is likely to be adversely affected by alcohol consumption. The lay public and medical community generally accept that alcohol impairs psychomotor performance in a dose-related manner. Perhaps we can best exemplify this assumption by the estimated increased fatality risk for drivers in single-vehicle crashes as the level of BAC increases. As figure 3.1 indicates, compared with nondrinking drivers, the risk of fatal injury was estimated to be 11.1 times greater for drivers with levels of BAC from .05 to .09, 48 times greater for drivers with levels of BAC from .10 to .14, and 385 times greater for drivers with levels of BAC at or above .15 (Zador, 1991).

Although it is widely accepted that the effects of alcohol on psychomotor performance are dose dependent, Manno and Manno (1988) indicated that this conclusion has been based on "seem-

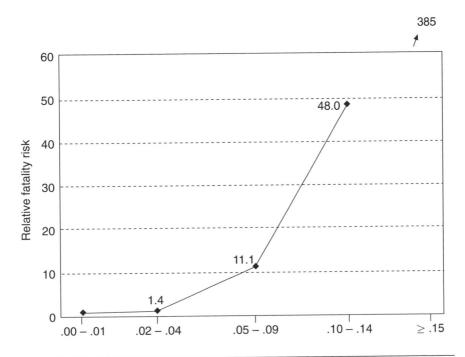

Figure 3.1 Estimated increased fatality risk for drivers in single-vehicle crashes at different levels of blood alcohol concentration (BAC).

From "Alcohol-Related Relative Risk of Fatal Driver Injuries in Relation to Driver Age and Sex" by P. L. Zador, 1991, *Journal of Studies on Alcohol, 52*, p. 302-310. Copyright 1991 by Alcohol Research Documentation, Inc., Rutgers Center of Alcohol Studies, Piscataway, NJ 08855. Adapted with permission.

ingly unrelated studies rather than through well-integrated scientific investigations" (p. 245). They further suggested that, because of the importance of documenting an accurate relationship between alcohol consumption and psychomotor performance, laboratory and field-based (including task simulation) studies testing this relationship are needed, in addition to the more frequent epidemiological studies.

The following sections will discuss conclusions from studies done in laboratory as well as in field settings to ascertain alcohol's impact on psychomotor performance. Keep in mind while reviewing these sections that the psychomotor skills needed for sport are not unlike the ones studied in the alcohol and human performance literature. Therefore, it is a reasonable assumption that sport skills will show alcohol-related changes similar to the following human performance measures.

Laboratory-Based Studies

Laboratory-based studies, where relevant variables may be precisely controlled, have confirmed an alcohol-related, dose-dependent performance impairment as measured by different sectors of psychomotor performance (i.e., sensory processing, central integration and processing mechanisms, overt motor responses, and overall sensory motor coordination [Hindmarch, 1980]). However, the diversity and number of tests used in different studies to measure the impact of alcohol on psychomotor performance have made comparisons between these studies difficult.

Even a cursory review of the literature on the alcohol and human performance relationship shows that numerous studies have examined a variety of independent and dependent variables. We can categorize the independent variables into environmental or subject variables. Environmental variables examined include dose of alcohol administered, time of administration, time delay between alcohol administration and performance task testing, performance testing during the ascending or descending limb of the blood alcohol curve, administration of other psychoactive drugs (e.g., nicotine), rate of ingestion of alcohol, paced and unpaced performance tasks, incentive instructions, and task difficulty. Examples of subject variables that have been manipulated include gender, body type as measured by fat content and weight, expectancy of alcohol effects, prior experience with alcohol, age, and introversion or extroversion.

Dependent variables have been numerous and often reflect an overlap between the skills tapped by each dependent measure. Some dependent measures used in studies include eye-hand coordination, reaction time (simple, complex, and choice), random number addition, body sway, divided attention, short-term memory, pursuit tracking ability, subjects' awareness of performance level, central processing of information, manual assembly tasks, standing and walking steadiness, and signal detection tasks.

Given the variety of independent and dependent variables that have been examined, it is difficult to make general conclusions about the alcohol-performance relationship. However, the finding that alcohol impairment on human performance is dose dependent appears to be consistent (Nuotto & Mattila, 1990). There are instances, however, in which low concentrations of alcohol may improve performance, perhaps because of tension-relieving properties of alcohol, particularly in tasks of short duration (Linnoila & Mattila, 1973). This phenomenon exemplifies the apparent biphasic effect of alcohol. In low concentrations, alcohol may stimulate various CNS functions by depressing inhibitory control mechanisms. As BAC increases, the CNS depressant effects are predominant.

In sum, laboratory-based studies suggest that alcohol does impair human performance dose dependently, with some exceptions at low BAC. Statistically significant effects found in the laboratory, however, do not necessarily translate to field settings. The next section will examine relationships found in field settings, including simulators.

Field Studies

Because impaired automobile driving has strong negative consequences for human morbidity and mortality, this psychomotor task has received considerable attention in field studies. Recent reviews (Howat, Sleet, & Smith, 1991; Moskowitz & Burns, 1990) have suggested that driving-related skills demonstrate decrements at levels of BAC of .05 or lower, although there is a wide inter-individual variation. Studies reviewed by Howat et al. were laboratory based as well as applied. Variables studied included visual and auditory simple and choice reaction time, visual vigilance, compensatory tracking, tracking with divided attention, driving simulation, car driving on circuit and on special maneuvers, and car driving in traffic experiments. Howat et al. argued in favor of lowering the legal limit of BAC to .05 in Australia where the study took place. Moscowitz and Burns (1990) suggested that the skills considered most important for safe driving—the "ability to observe, interpret, and process information from the eyes and other senses . . ." (p. 14)—are particularly vulnerable to the effects of alcohol even at BAC levels of .01 to .02, the lowest that can be measured reliably.

The effects of alcohol on performance of pilots also has been a subject of study, again because of the potential disastrous results of impaired performance. Collins (1980) found that a BAC of approximately .09 yielded performance decrements in simulated flight tasks. In particular, Collins found that acute alcohol ingestion resulted in impaired tracking performance and visual reaction time; however, no performance decrements were noted on tasks performed approximately eight hours after drinking (hangover condition). Yesavage and Leirer (1986) also studied the delayed effects of alcohol on flight-related tasks. They found that there were hangover effects on pilot performance in simulated flights 14 hours after ingesting alcohol sufficient to obtain a BAC of .10. Collins indicated that his results offered no contraindications to the *eight-hour rule,* which prohibits pilots from flying within eight hours of drinking alcohol. However, Collins suggested that results should be interpreted cautiously because subjects were well motivated and interested in the outcome of the research, and common aviator stressors such as engine noise were not present. On the other hand, Yesavage and Leirer concluded that pilots should exercise caution when flying aircraft 14 hours or less after ingesting alcohol sufficient to produce a BAC of .10. Additional controlled studies are needed to make firm conclusions about the time needed to eliminate the effects of varying dosages of alcohol on performance.

In sum, field studies indicate detrimental effects of alcohol on performance, although specific levels of BAC needed to yield performance decrements vary across individuals. Recent reviews of the effects of alcohol on driving performance (Moscowitz & Burns, 1990; Howat et al., 1991) suggested that impairment is being found at lower BAC levels than noted previously. Indeed, Howat et al. suggested that there is sufficient scientific evidence to decrease the legal BAC for driving to .05, a level where most people's driving performance is impaired. Most states in the United States have .10 as the legal limit for intoxication. Some states have recently changed that limit to .08 and many states are considering similar legislation.

What do the results of these studies on human performance effects of alcohol mean for the athlete? Essentially, they indicate that, to the extent athletic skills depend on the same psychomotor skills examined in these studies, athletic performance will suffer. As a rule, the more complex the skills required by a particular sport, the more alcohol-related decrements in performance we can expect. Furthermore, the less practiced (or less automatic) the skill, the more likely alcohol will negatively affect performance, as suggested in reviews by Howat et al. (1991).

The following section describes research that documents the effects of alcohol on sport performance. As you read it, keep in mind the findings of studies already mentioned about the effects of alcohol on various human performance measures.

ERGOLYTIC AND ERGOGENIC EFFECTS OF ALCOHOL ON SPORT PERFORMANCE

In the late 1800s alcohol was reportedly used to enhance sport performance (i.e., as an ergogenic aid). Boje (as cited in Williams, 1991) indicated that, in athletic situations of extreme exertion or in events requiring brief maximal effort, alcohol has been given to athletes as a stimulant to release inhibitions and decrease sense of fatigue. Jokl (1968) reported widespread alcohol use in European athletics at the turn of the century. He reported incidents of marathon runners consuming large quantities of cognac during competition and cyclists consuming rum and champagne throughout 24-hour races. The apparent rationale for alcohol consumption was to refresh the athlete and restore their strength. Pistol shooters have used alcohol as a supposed ergogenic to decrease anxiety levels, allowing maximum performance. Before 1968, the use of alcohol was proscribed as a doping agent by the International Olympic Committee (IOC), and two pistol shooters were disqualified in the 1968 Olympics because of alleged alcohol use (Shephard, 1972). During the 1972 Munich Olympics, however, alcohol was not included on the list of outlawed doping agents (Fischbach, as cited in Williams, 1991). This despite the fact that athletes involved in shooting competitions referred to alcohol as "goldwater."

Although historically athletes have used alcohol to improve sport performance, more recent evidence indicates that alcohol rarely is an ergogenic aid and in most cases detracts from athletic performance (i.e., has ergolytic effects). In its position stand on alcohol use in sport, the American College of Sports Medicine (ACSM, 1982) concluded the following about the acute ingestion of alcohol:

1. Alcohol in small (1.5 to 2.0 oz) to moderate (3 to 4 oz) amounts has negative effects on a variety of psychomotor skills, including reaction time, eye-hand coordination, accuracy, balance, and complex coordination or gross motor skills.

2. Alcohol apparently has little or no beneficial effects on metabolic or physiological functions underlying physical performance (e.g., energy metabolism and functions that contribute to oxygen consumption and maximal oxygen consumption, heart rate, stroke volume, cardiac output).

Furthermore, in those studies demonstrating significant effects, changes appear to decrease performance. Alcohol may adversely affect body temperature regulation during prolonged exercise in cold temperatures.

3. Alcohol will not improve and potentially may decrease muscular work capacity.

In addition to this list, the ACSM position stand indicated that alcohol is the most abused drug in the United States and is a contributing factor to accidents. Also noted is the negative impact of prolonged excessive use of alcohol on major organ systems of the body (e.g., liver, heart, brain, and muscle). The ACSM called for continued efforts to educate athletes, coaches, and sport-related professionals, as well as the general public, about the effects of alcohol on human performance and the potential negative consequences of long-term excessive alcohol use. The following sections will address the three areas in the ACSM position stand regarding the effects of acute alcohol ingestion on athletic performance and the effects of social drinking as a lifestyle choice.

Psychomotor Effects

Although alcohol consumption may be seductive for athletes as a mechanism to positively influence psychological well-being and performance, evidence suggests that alcohol is likely to impair psychomotor skills essential to sport performance. Coopersmith (1964) noted, based on anthropological and clinical evidence as well as popular conception, that small amounts of alcohol reduce feelings of insecurity and tension, permitting a freer expression of behavior. Related to this observation, it has been suggested that alcohol may strengthen the athlete's self-confidence (Shephard, 1972). More recent evidence, however, indicates that the risks for a decline in psychomotor skills associated with alcohol consumption outweigh the potential benefits of alcohol on tension level or self-confidence for most individuals. Literature reviewed previously in this chapter indicated that deficits in psychomotor skills may occur at levels of BAC of .05 or less. Although there is considerable variation in susceptibility among individuals to the psychomotor effects of alcohol, complex skills requiring central processing capacity are usually impaired at lower BAC levels (Mitchell, 1985). For example, Moskowitz, Burns, and Williams (1985) found that psychomotor tasks involving divided attention, tracking, visual search, recognition and response were impaired with levels of BAC as low as .015. Conversely, Mitchell noted that other psychomotor skills, such as simple reaction time, may show no or little deficits at levels of BAC approaching .10. Therefore, the effects of alcohol on psychomotor performance appear to be mediated by negative effects on central processing capabilities (Baylor, Layne, Mayfield, Osborne, & Spirduso, 1989).

Because alcohol has significant antianxiety and antitremor effects (Koller & Biary, 1984), alcohol consumption may positively affect performance in sports requiring steady hands and aim, such as pistol shooting and archery. Research in this area is scarce and inconclusive. For example, Reilly and Halliday (1985) found differential effects of alcohol (levels of BAC at .02 and .05) on tasks related to archery such that arm steadiness deteriorated and reaction time slowed at both BAC levels (possible impairments) and release was smoother at .02 (possible enhancement). No effects of alcohol were shown on strength or endurance. Unfortunately, performance data were not reported, so judgment regarding ergogenic effects was not possible. Even though research is inconclusive regarding alcohol's ergogenic effects on performance in precision shooting sports, its use is banned in these competitive activities based on its known antianxiety effects.

Effects on Metabolic and Physiological Functions Underlying Sport Performance

The position stand of the ACSM is that alcohol appears to have little or no beneficial effect on metabolic and physiological functions important to physical performance. Furthermore, in those studies reviewed in the ACSM position stand that indicated a significant effect of alcohol on performance, the effect was detrimental.

Studies since the ACSM position stand in 1982 have essentially corroborated its conclusions. For example, Heikkonen (1989) found that acute alcohol intake had minor negative effects on exercise-induced changes in hormonal and metabolic activity in young healthy male subjects. This researcher reported, among other findings, that physical exercise intensified and prolonged alcohol's depressant effect on testosterone production; that alcohol consumption immediately before or after exercise reduced the human growth hormone secretion increase normally found following exercise; and alcohol taken immediately before exercise inhibited the typical exercise-induced increase in blood glucose levels and therefore caused mild hypoglycemia during the recovery phase from exercise after fasting. Interestingly, this hypoglycemic effect also was observed after exercise during hangover. Other studies using the bicycle ergometer test similarly showed that alcohol had no beneficial effects on metabolic or work performance measures (Bond, Franks, & Howley, 1984; Borg, Domserius, & Kaijser, 1990). Borg et al. also reported that moderate doses of alcohol did not alter subjects' perceived exertion. Mangum, Gatch, Cocke, and Brooks (1986) found that beer had no obvious benefit as a replacement fluid during submaximal exercise on a bicycle ergometer. This result calls into question the belief of some exercisers that beer would be advantageous as a replacement fluid.

Although studies since the ACSM position stand have confirmed that alcohol has no beneficial effects on metabolic and physiological responses to exercise, there have been occasional results that are inconsistent with this conclusion. For example, Amusa and Muoboghare (1986) found differing effects of alcohol on physiological processes in response to exercise. They studied the effects of three levels of BAC (.03, .05, .10) on various physical performance parameters. They found no effect of alcohol on resting blood pressure or on exercise-related blood pressure, heart rate, and oxygen uptake. However, they found that alcohol at the dosages used in the experiment increased the resting heart rate, work duration, and recovery heart rate. These authors speculated that the apparent positive effect of alcohol on work duration is mediated by its effect on resting heart rate, which may reduce fatigue, or by its inhibitory effect on the brain, thereby reducing perception of fatigue. Although this is an interesting speculation, there is limited support for this hypothesis.

Effects on Tests of Fitness Components

Similar to its findings regarding the effects of alcohol on the metabolic and physiological functions underlying performance, the ACSM concluded that alcohol will not improve muscular work capacity and may lead to decreases in performance levels. Studies cited in the ACSM position stand indicated alcohol may decrease dynamic muscular strength, isometric grip strength, dynamometer strength, power, and ergographic muscular output. Other studies cited by ACSM indicated no effect of alcohol on muscular strength, local muscular endurance, physical performance capacity, exercise time at maximum levels, or exercise time to exhaustion.

A representative sample of more recent studies substantiates ACSM conclusions in 1982. Bond, Gresham, Balkissoon, and Clearwater (1984) found no effect of small (.34 g/kg body weight) or moderate (.69 g/kg body weight) amounts of alcohol on peak and average torque-generating capabilities during elbow flexion and extension and knee extension. McNaughton and Preece (1986) concluded that alcohol in different amounts had no ergogenic properties for performances in the 100-, 200-, 400-, 800-, and 1500-m track events. Alcohol negatively affected all events to varying degrees, except the 100-m event, which remained stable. Finally, Houmard, Langenfeld, Wiley, and Siefert (1987) found no significant differences in performances on the 5-mile treadmill for 18 well-trained male runners who consumed either low levels (BAC level less than .05) or no alcohol. The authors concluded that alcohol ingestion yielding low levels of BAC does not enhance performance of endurance exercise.

SOCIAL DRINKING AND SPORT PERFORMANCE

Although numerous studies have investigated the acute effects of alcohol consumption on sport performance, given drinking incidence among athletes, an important issue for most athletes and coaches is the effects of social drinking on performance, specifically, its potential cumulative effects on fitness levels and its effects on performance if alcohol consumption occurs the night before a competition.

With respect to the first issue, the effect of social drinking on fitness, epidemiological data, although inconsistent, suggest that alcohol consumption in moderation has neither beneficial nor detrimental effects on physical performance (see review by Williams, 1991). The second issue, performance decrements following alcohol consumption the previous night, relates to the amount of alcohol consumed. Although this area has received limited research attention, it appears that light drinking the night before will not significantly influence physical performance the following morning. For example, MacDonald and Svoboda (as cited in Williams, 1991) found that one drink consumed nightly for 10 days had no significant effects on measures involving strength, power, and aerobic exercise performed the following morning. Heavier drinking, however, may yield different results. Karvinin, Miettinen, and Ahlman (1962) found that consuming an average of 1.67 grams of alcohol per kilogram of body weight (about eight drinks in this study) did not significantly influence performance on tests of static strength or power the following morning, but apparently hampered aerobic performance. In a more recent study, O'Brien (1993) found significant decrements in aerobic performance of rugby players following alcohol consumption of varying amounts the previous night; however, no effects of alcohol were found on anaerobic performance. Also of interest in this study is the individual variability players demonstrated in their susceptibility to the next-day effects of alcohol on aerobic performance. Some players showed sensitivity to the aftereffects of alcohol consumption the night before and demonstrated significant decrements in aerobic performance after small amounts of alcohol relative to some of their peers. Conversely, other players drank substantially more alcohol and suffered equal, and in some cases less, aerobic performance decreases the following morning than their more alcohol-susceptible peers.

Another important issue about social drinking is the diuretic effect of alcohol (Williams, 1991). It is not uncommon for some athletes to consume alcohol the night before competition or following an endurance event such as the marathon. Because alcohol has diuretic properties, consumption before an endurance event, or any event in which there is significant fluid loss through sweating, may cause dehydration with adverse performance effects. Also, an athlete consuming alcohol after such an event, in a state of dehydration and with an empty stomach, would be susceptible to a rapid absorption and concentration of alcohol in the body. Because even small amounts of alcohol impair psychomotor skills, it is particularly unwise for a dehydrated athlete to drink alcohol and attempt to drive an automobile or do any potentially dangerous task requiring psychomotor skills.

CONCLUSION

In reviewing the biomedical and behavioral effects of alcohol, it comes as no surprise that alcohol has the potential to significantly influence human functioning. Acute effects of alcohol on the central nervous system substantiate the findings that alcohol impairs psychomotor performance dependent on dose. Prolonged heavy drinking carries with it, in addition to the risk of addiction, the risk of serious physical and behavioral consequences as reviewed in the chapter.

The sport literature, typified by the ACSM position stand, concludes that alcohol does not have ergogenic characteristics for any sport applications. Although alcohol may yield some performance-enhancing effects on sports such as pistol shooting and archery, which may be disrupted by excessive anxiety, available evidence is ambiguous. However, the use of alcohol in conjunction with these competitions is banned based on its known antianxiety effects. The effects of alcohol appear to be most disruptive in sports that require complex psychomotor skills. Other sport-related functions (e.g., metabolic and physiological processes, muscular work capacity) show little or no beneficial effects in response to alcohol or show decrements. Social drinking is generally not regarded as ergolytic. However, excessive consumption the night before a morning competition may adversely affect performance.

Given the conclusion that alcohol at best yields no ergogenic effects for most sports, what are the recommendations for athletes about drinking? The ACSM position stand offers the following:

> *Serious and continuing efforts should be made to educate athletes, coaches, health and physical educators, physicians, trainers, the sports media, and the general public regarding the effects of acute alcohol ingestion upon human physical performance and on the potential acute and chronic problems of excessive alcohol consumption. (ACSM, 1982, p. ix)*

A variety of articles can be found in the popular sport and coaching literature over the last 20 years that contribute to this educational effort (e.g., Coleman, 1989; Dickinson, 1979; Harvey, 1991; Hoffman, 1977; Leyshon, 1976; Masia, 1978; Mirkin, 1981; Porterfield, 1987; "Puff, Puff," 1982; Salo, 1988; Smith, 1979; Tanny, 1986; Wynd, 1988). The ACSM recommends a guideline based on Anstie's rule (as cited in ACSM, 1982) for moderate, safe drinking for adults. This rule defines safe drinking levels as up to .5 oz of pure alcohol per 23 kg (51 lb) of body weight per day. This is the equivalent of three bottles of beer

(4.2 percent alcohol), three 4-oz glasses of 13 percent wine, or 3 oz of 50 percent whiskey for a 68-kg (150-lb) person. Although this is a recommended guideline, it does not take into account individual differences in responses to alcohol. All individuals carry various risks for alcohol abuse in their genetic makeup and life experiences (see section on risk factors in chapter 1). We must not neglect this fact when considering safe levels of drinking.

4 ALCOHOL ABUSE AND DEPENDENCE AMONG ATHLETES AND SPORT PROFESSIONALS

That poignant liquor, which the zealot calls the mother
of sins, is pleasant and sweet to me. Give me wine!
Wine that shall subdue the strongest, that I may for
a time forget the cares and troubles of the world.

—Anonymous

We will now turn our attention to alcohol abuse and dependence among athletes and sport professionals. This chapter contains sections on the incidence of and risk factors for alcohol-related disorders in these populations. A major portion of the chapter presents case studies, giving the reader descriptive, representative scenarios of athletes, coaches, and sport-related health professionals with alcohol problems. The chapter concludes with a summary of issues and diagnostic considerations relevant to the case studies. Coaches and a sport-related health professional are included in the case studies because these professionals identify and intervene with athletes who have alcohol problems. If these professionals are experiencing similar problems, it will probably hamper their ability to assist athletes. Therefore, readers should remember the potentially significant role they can play, not only in recognizing alcohol-related problems among athletes, but also among colleagues. Successful intervention with a colleague experiencing alcohol-related problems enhances that person's life and professional effectiveness, which ultimately will increase his or her ability to serve athletes.

INCIDENCE OF ALCOHOL ABUSE AND DEPENDENCE AMONG ATHLETES

The limited data available on incidence of alcohol abuse and dependence among athletes suggest that the frequency of these problems approximates and may exceed general population estimates (approximately 9 percent of the over age 18 population in 1988 met DSM-III-R diagnostic criteria for alcohol abuse or dependence [Grant, Harford, et al., 1991]). For example, in a survey of high school, college, and professional athletes, Heitzinger and Associates (1986) indicated that 6.5 percent of high school athletes, 5 percent of college athletes, and 26 percent of professional athletes reported receiving counseling for alcohol or drug problems. This data is confounded by inclusion of drug use, making it impossible to determine incidence of alcohol abuse and dependence alone. Also, it cannot be assumed that receiving counseling or treatment means the individual's alcohol use met diagnostic criteria for alcohol abuse or dependence. Conversely, it could be argued that these estimates are conservative given that many individuals potentially meeting diagnostic criteria for alcohol abuse or dependence do not seek treatment and are not recognized as alcohol abusers when being treated for other health problems.

Even though research documenting the incidence of alcohol abuse and dependence among athletes is scarce, there is no lack of anecdotal reports suggesting that alcohol and drug abuse or dependence are a matter of concern. An article in *The Sporting News* (Nightingale, 1981) suggested that management in many professional sport leagues was concerned about the level of alcohol and drug use or abuse. The following quotes from that article document this concern.

> 'There isn't a team in the major leagues, ours included, that doesn't have an alcohol problem.' (Ballard Smith, President, San Diego Padres [p. 13])

> Anyone who attempts to put a quantification on chemical abuse by athletes, or by society as a whole, is kidding himself. . . . But we do have a problem and I perceive our problem is getting worse. Society has a problem, and we are a mirror of society . . . except that we must be aware we have a higher visibility than society. (Bowie Kuhn, Commissioner of Major League Baseball [p. 13])

> It is naive to think we don't have drug users in our league . . . But I must confess I don't know the depths of any problems we might have with alcoholism. Alcohol presents us, and any sport, with a special problem. We can tell our athletes they can't use drugs which are illegal. But how can we tell them they can't use something (alcohol) that is legal? (Frank Torpey, Chief Security Officer for the National Hockey League [p. 13])

> Cocaine, marijuana, and amphetamines, in that order, are the three things that cause us the most concern . . . and, yet, alcoholism may be our No. 1 problem. (Warren Welsh, Chief Security Officer for the National Football League [p. 13])

The number of high-profile athletes who have come forth describing their alcohol abuse and dependence problems, although not clarifying the overall incidence of alcohol abuse in professional sport, certainly indicates that high-level athletes are not immune to developing alcohol-related problems. The list of athletes describing alcohol abuse or alcohol dependence in their lives is long and includes representatives from a variety of sports: Dennis Eckersley (Krentzman, 1991), Mickey Mantle (Mantle & Lieber, 1994), and Bob Welch (Fimrite, 1990; Welch & Vecsey, 1982) in baseball; John Lucas (Lieber, 1993) and Lloyd Daniels (Valenti & Naclerio, 1990) in basketball; Carol Mann (Byrd,

1991b) and John Daly (Reilly, 1993) in golf; Tai Babilonia (Byrd, 1991b) in ice skating; Derek Sanderson (Byrd, 1991b) in ice hockey; and Dexter Manley (Reilly, 1987) in football. This list is only a small sample of the many athletes that have been willing to share their personal stories of difficulties with alcohol. Although most of these athletes developed their alcohol abuse over years, the effects of alcohol were swiftly and tragically introduced in some lives. In spring training of 1993, Cleveland Indian pitchers Tim Crews and Steve Olin lost their lives in an alcohol-related boating accident (Smith, 1993). Similarly, Bill Shoemaker, a highly decorated jockey, was rendered a quadriplegic following an alcohol-related automobile accident (Nack, 1993). Lenny Dykstra and Darren Daulton of the Philadelphia Phillies also were involved in an alcohol-related automobile accident, which resulted in injuries to both players ("Live and Learn," 1991). These three incidences of alcohol-related tragedy attest that one does not have to be an identified alcoholic to suffer consequences of alcohol use.

RISK FACTORS FOR ALCOHOL ABUSE AND DEPENDENCE AMONG ATHLETES

Although athletes do not exhibit a higher incidence of alcohol abuse and dependence than the general population, they may have risk factors in common with the general population and risk factors related to their participation in sport. Like the general population, athletes can be at greater risk for alcohol abuse and dependence if they have a family history of alcoholism (Tarter & Edwards, 1986). The extent to which this increased risk is based on biological or psychosocial variables is still a matter of scientific debate. A recent study by Sweeney (1987/1988) indicated that the best predictor of alcohol misuse among collegiate football players was psychological health of one's family of origin. The study found that athletes from psychologically troubled families not only exhibited a propensity to misuse alcohol but also tended toward negative mood states such as anger and depression. Conversely, athletes from psychologically healthy families were not inclined toward alcohol misuse nor were they angry, depressed, confused, tense, or fatigued. They also tended to be successful athletes. This study suggested that athletes, just as the general population, are susceptible to mental health and family-of-origin risk factors for alcohol abuse.

An important question about risk factors for athletes is whether the experience of athletic participation carries with it unique risk factors for alcohol abuse (environmental risk factors) or whether those individuals drawn to sport bring with them characteristics placing them at increased risk (individual risk factors). These etiologically different factors (one emanating from the sport experience and the other from the athlete) are difficult to tease apart. It is likely that one or both factors play a role in the risk of an athlete experiencing problems with alcohol. Nattiv and Puffer (1991) surveyed intercollegiate athletes and nonathletes about lifestyle and health risk behaviors and found that a significantly higher proportion of athletes reported risky lifestyle behavioral patterns in the following areas: quantity of alcohol consumption, driving while intoxicated on alcohol or drugs, riding with an intoxicated driver, seat belt use, use of helmets when riding a motorcycle or moped, use of contraception, number of sexually transmitted diseases, and number of sexual partners. Although it is not possible from this study to determine whether participation in sport or individual inclinations of athletes not related to sport participation are responsible for these risky behaviors, it is significant that, relative to their nonathlete peers, collegiate athletes are placing themselves at higher risk for alcohol-related and other problems with their lifestyle choices.

In a recent review article, Tricker, Cook, and McGuire (1989) discussed a number of hypotheses regarding how the sport experience may place college athletes at greater risk for alcohol or drug abuse. Many risks directly relate to the rewards and frustrations of athletic competition. Athletes are expected to maintain high levels of performance, often in the face of tremendous stressors. They are under constant scrutiny by friends, family, the media, and the general public, and consequently their successes and failures are on public display. The expectations placed on athletes frequently are beyond their developmental level of accomplishment. Therefore, they may consistently feel pressure to improve their skills at a rate that is not self-determined. The lifestyle of the athlete is often characterized by travel and exposure to social settings that frequently include the use of alcohol if not other drugs. Exposure to these settings may occur at a pace that outstrips the social skills development needed for the athlete to adapt to this lifestyle. Combined with the need to adapt to a new social world are the emotional highs and lows of athletic competition. Alcohol use may become an attractive coping mechanism to handle these social and sport-related pressures. This may be particularly the case because athletes are often separated from more traditional support, such as family and close friends.

As indicated by the Nattiv and Puffer (1991) study, college athletes may be prone to high-risk behavior, including alcohol abuse. This tendency, along with superior levels of physical prowess, may encourage athletes to see themselves as not susceptible or possibly invulnerable to the effects of alcohol. In addition, their youthful vigor may allow them to continue performing athletically despite increasing alcohol use, which when combined with tendencies to minimize risks associated with alcohol use, can make early diagnosis of alcoholism difficult (Chappell, 1987).

Finally, retirement from an athletic career may present significant problems for the athlete (Ogilvie, 1987). After leading an atypical lifestyle of practice and competition, the athlete faces the prospect of life after sport. For many, the adjustment is difficult, because few life experiences can parallel the intensity and excitement of athletic competition. For some, alcohol use may be an inviting replacement for the lost excitement of their careers or a way to self-medicate the pains associated with the transition to a new lifestyle.

Just as their collegiate counterparts experience sport-related risk factors for alcohol abuse, high school athletes also experience risk factors for alcohol abuse related to their athletic participation, as suggested by Good (1985). These risk factors might include environmental pressures such as negative role modeling by professional athletes; peer pressure involved in team membership if other team members are using alcohol; sacrifices demanded by coaches; and parents', friends', and teachers' expectations for the athlete's performance. Other risk factors for high school athletes relate to developmental tasks associated with adolescence, which may or may not relate to sport. These include defining a healthy identity, developing a mature sexuality, dealing with success and failure associated with athletic participation, coping with injury, and developing intellectually when the demands of school often conflict with the demands of sport. Added to these potential risk factors for alcohol abuse is the fact that most adolescent athletes will be facing retirement from their competitive sport either in high school or college. For those athletes who have not established other competencies and identities, this abrupt transition to retirement from sport will be difficult, and the likelihood of alcohol abuse will increase.

Although risk factors for alcohol abuse in male and female adolescent athletes may be similar, they differ with regard to developing a mature sexuality. For boys, the risk comes primarily from the notion that being a successful athlete is associated with being able to "hold one's liquor." The countless alcohol-related commercials that associate sport and alcohol consumption reinforce this connection. For young female athletes, the issue of dealing with a potential sex role conflict may underlie an increased risk for alcohol abuse. A recent study by Wetzig (1990) with female college athletes and female alcoholics in treatment found that they were similar to each other and different from female undergraduate students in various dimensions of sex role conflict, including feminine socialization, power needs, competition, and sensation seeking. The author suggested that both female athletes and alcoholics experience conflict between traditionally male stereotype traits of assertion, independence, and achievement and more traditionally feminine traits of dependence and affiliation. With the increased availability of athletic opportunities for women, perhaps this sex role conflict, which may place female athletes at higher risk for alcohol abuse, will diminish.

INCIDENCE OF ALCOHOL ABUSE AND DEPENDENCE AMONG SPORT PROFESSIONALS

Because of the scarcity of literature on alcohol abuse and dependence among coaches, general population estimates are the only reasonable figures from which to generalize to this subpopulation.

Unlike for coaches, there are significant reports in the literature regarding the incidence of alcohol abuse and dependence among health professionals, particularly physicians and nurses. For example, in a survey of faculty and house staff physicians at an urban, university-based teaching hospital, Siegel and Fitzgerald (1988) found that 4 percent of respondents were classified as alcoholic and 10 percent possibly alcoholic as measured by a modified version of the Short Michigan Alcoholic Screening Test (a self-administered questionnaire frequently used to screen for alcoholism). A similar study (Lewy, 1986) done with house staff physicians at a New York City medical center found a rate of 12.7 percent of respondents having scores on the self-administered version of the Michigan Alcoholism Screening Test indicating either suspicion or presumption of alcoholism. A recent review (Sullivan & Handley, 1992) of alcohol and drug abuse among nurses concluded that nurses do not experience these problems exceeding societal rates. Another study (Trinkoff, Eaton, & Anthony, 1991) suggested that nurses may be less likely to have alcohol-abuse problems than non-nurses. Regardless of the estimated incidence of these conditions among health professionals, their mere presence in this occupational group is troubling in that the work performed by these professionals is so important to the health and well-being of their patients.

In addition to prevalence studies there are descriptive and anecdotal reports that provide important information about alcohol abuse and dependence among health professionals. For instance, Tipliski (1993) described characteristics of chemically dependent nurses. She found that among other characteristics these nurses reported a high divorce rate, a family history of chemical dependence and depressive illness, multiple traumatic sexual events, occupational stress, and initiation of drug abuse through self-medication. Similarly, Bissell and Skorina (1987) interviewed alcoholic, female physicians and medical students to gain some insight into this population. They found that addiction to multiple drugs in addition to alcohol was common, along with suicidal ideation and attempts, marital instability, and presence of alcoholics in the nuclear family. Recognizing the importance of intervening with chemically dependent health professionals, many states have committees charged with implementing mechanisms to identify impaired health professionals and to encourage them to seek treatment. Often this encouragement includes the threat of loss of license to practice. Among nurses, it has been emphasized that it is the responsibility of the entire profession to ensure that programs are in place in all states to educate nurses regarding chemical dependence and to assist impaired nurses needing treatment for this condition or related problems (Green, 1989).

RISK FACTORS FOR ALCOHOL ABUSE AND DEPENDENCE AMONG SPORT PROFESSIONALS

Just as for athletes, sport professionals have risk factors for alcohol abuse and dependence that are in common with the general population and factors unique to their professions. Because many individuals reaching the coaching ranks are former or current competitive athletes, we can expect that coaches will have experienced the athletically oriented risk factors for alcohol abuse. Most pressures experienced by athletes continue to be part of coaches' work situations, and some of these pressures may be magnified. Coaches face similar challenges as parents in that they may prepare athletes as best as possible for competition but are unable to play the game for the athlete. Hence, there may be a feeling of limited control, not only of athletes in competition but also of their longevity as coaches. In addition, depending on the individual coach's situation, the demands of recruiting; practice; reacting to athlete issues; budget planning; supervising assistant coaches; and dealing effectively with parents, alumni, school administration, and fans contribute to the complexity and stress associated with the coaching profession. Alcohol, because of its tranquilizing properties, may provide relief from these stressors and, in the vulnerable individual, lead to overreliance on a chemical solution for problems.

As with coaches, health professionals may use alcohol or other drugs to assist them in dealing with demanding careers. Many health professionals endure extended postgraduate education, often under stressful conditions with limited or nonexistent emotional support to help them cope effectively. In the case of physicians, certain psychological motivations to study medicine, as well as the emotionally punishing nature of medical education, combine to make physicians in training susceptible to mental health problems, including alcohol and drug abuse (Johnson, 1991). The same may be true, although to a lesser extent, for nurses. Also, education regarding alcohol and drug abuse is noticeably absent or diminished relative to other topics.

A recent study by Moore, Mead, and Pearson (1990) indicated numerous medical school precursors associated with subsequent alcohol abuse in male physicians. A partial list of these precursors includes lack of religious affiliation, regular use of alcohol, a history of alcohol-related difficulty, and cigarette use of one pack or more per day. Although this study is correlational and therefore cannot provide a basis for statements about causes of physician alcohol abuse, it provides clues for development of alcohol abuse in this population.

Two factors that contribute to alcohol and drug abuse among health professionals are so-called pharmacologic optimism and easy access to mind-altering drugs (Crosby & Bissell, 1989). Pharmacologic optimism refers to the belief that medications are a panacea for all problems. Health professionals have high-level knowledge of drug actions and may underestimate their vulnerability to addiction. They also may labor under the false impression that their knowledge of drugs will in some way protect them from chemical dependency. Therefore, their education may be a liability for their risk for addiction.

A second risk factor unique to health professionals is easy access to mind-altering drugs. Although alcohol is easily accessible to the general population, prescription drugs with similar properties are much more accessible to the health professional. Many of these drugs are cross-tolerant with alcohol, which means that while one develops tolerance to a prescription drug such as Valium, a concomitant tolerance is developed to alcohol. Therefore, when one drug is unavailable the other may be used as a substitute. The health professional who acquires an addiction to prescription drugs may subsequently or simultaneously develop an addiction to alcohol.

Finally, the stresses associated with a career in medicine, nursing, or allied health professions may contribute to risk for alcohol or drug abuse. A study by Sutherland and Cooper (1993), examining predictors of illness and job dissatisfaction among general practitioners, found that male doctors exhibited significantly higher levels of anxiety and depression than a normative sample, whereas female doctors were similar to population norms. Primary predictors of lack of mental health were the stressors related to job demands and patients' expectations, practice administration and routine medical work, role stress, and low use of social support as a coping mechanism. This study suggests that health professionals become more vulnerable to alcohol abuse when they have difficulty adapting successfully to these job-related stressors.

CASE STUDIES: DESCRIPTION AND DIAGNOSTIC ANALYSIS

This section contains clinical case vignettes describing athletes and sport professionals with problems related to their alcohol consumption, including alcohol abuse or dependence. These vignettes are an amalgamation of case material and anecdotal information intended for instructional purposes to demonstrate salient features of individuals with alcohol-related problems. A discussion of relevant clinical issues will follow each case description.

Alcohol-Abusing Athletes

The following vignettes describe two athletes experiencing problems associated with their alcohol consumption. When reading the vignettes, pay particular attention to behavioral characteristics associated with alcohol-related problems. Also, remember that alcohol abuse and dependence differ primarily in the degree of severity of symptoms; these disorders are on a continuum of severity from less (alcohol abuse) to more (alcohol dependence) severe.

CASE STUDY

Donna

Donna was a 19-year-old college basketball player referred by her athletic trainer. On the intake interview, she indicated that she was not sure why her athletic trainer referred her for an appointment. She stated that she was a freshman and recently had sustained a knee injury that ended her participation in basketball for her freshman year. She said that the injury was a great disappointment for her because she was having an excellent year and contributing to the team. When questioned about her athletic history, Donna stated that she participated in both softball and basketball in high school and had an opportunity to play both sports at the college level. She reported that high school was fun for her, and she considered those years to be normal. She had a good relationship with both her parents and neither had histories of mental health or substance abuse problems. When questioned about her alcohol and drug use while in high school, she admitted that she took "a drink or two" but she did not consider her use a problem for her. She denied any drug use.

Donna said that her adjustment to college had been adequate initially, but much more difficult since her injury. Her friends apparently had been limited to teammates, but recently she had met other people she liked and had been spending time with them. Her recovery from the knee injury had been slow, but Donna stated that she had been following the rehabilitation plan to the best of her ability (her athletic trainer reported that she had been inconsistent in her compliance with the rehabilitation regimen). Donna reported that since her injury she had not felt like being around her teammates, even though she was required to go to practices and games. Her academic performance was apparently much lower than she expected based on her grades in high school. Donna reported that since her injury she had begun to meet new friends and was doing a lot more "partying." Although her drinking was significantly greater than when she was in high school, she did not perceive it to be a problem. She indicated that she usually went to one or two parties a week and typically drank "enough to get a buzz." She couldn't clarify how much alcohol she drank to get the desired effect. She stated that her drinking had increased primarily because she was hanging out with a different crowd, but when questioned further, she admitted that she occasionally drank to "forget about my injury." Ensuing sessions with Donna revealed that she had withdrawn from her teammates, her academic performance had decreased since her injury, and her coach had expressed concern about her slow recovery and her disinclination to be involved with her teammates.

DIAGNOSTIC SUMMARY

A number of issues are important to notice in Donna's situation. Her history suggests that she was a typical adolescent in high school, aside from being an exceptional athlete. She reported occasional experimentation with alcohol while in high school, which is a common practice for American adolescents. Upon entry into college, she was handling the rigors of the student-athlete lifestyle adequately until she was injured during the early part of the season. Her injury was associated with several troubling behavioral changes. She had withdrawn from her teammates; she had begun new friendships, which related to an increase in her frequency and intensity of drinking; her academic performance had suffered; and she had been inconsistent in complying with her rehabilitation regimen. This cluster of behavioral changes suggests that Donna was having difficulty coping and perhaps was using alcohol as a mechanism to handle her problems. Although her drinking level was difficult to ascertain with this history and perhaps did not meet the DSM-IV diagnostic criteria for alcohol abuse, her use of alcohol as a coping mechanism was reason for concern.

Although additional information about Donna's drinking is needed, her history suggests that her alcohol use had been prompted by several environmental stressors. These included adjustment to the social and academic demands of the college athlete and a season-ending injury from which she was recovering slowly. She apparently had been through a difficult rehabilitation process and had not complied with recommended rehabilitation activities. Also, she had withdrawn from teammates, a potential source of support during her recovery. Her history did not indicate any strong risk factors for developing alcohol abuse or dependence, which is a positive prognostic sign.

CASE STUDY

Mike

Mike was a 21-year-old college senior playing on the football team whose coach referred him following several incidents, including missing curfews, arguing with teammates, and disagreeing with coaching staff. In addition, Mike had recently had his second arrest in the last six months for driving under the influence (DUI) and was facing fines as well as prolonged legal sanctions to his license. He was currently suspended from football participation indefinitely.

During an initial session, Mike was reticent to talk, appeared angry, and voiced his resentment about having to come to the appointment. He didn't understand why his coaches and teammates felt something was wrong with him, even though he understood their concern about his violating team rules, his legal problems, and his argumentativeness. When questioned about his typical levels of alcohol intake, Mike chuckled and said he didn't drink any more than the average college student. He stated that he enjoyed drinking beer, and he and his friends would usually go out on weekends to "have some fun." He felt his most recent DUI charge was unlucky and that he really had not had much to drink that night (the police report indicated Mike's BAC was .15, which is substantially over the legal limit of .10). When asked about other drug use, Mike was evasive and stated that he had experimented with several other drugs during high school and college but declined to discuss it further. Mike's academic performance while in college had been inconsistent, which was similar to his performance in high school. Mike originated from a family of five, with two brothers, one of whom was a cocaine abuser and was now apparently abstinent from cocaine after treatment. His father had significant problems with alcohol and had recently quit drinking after inpatient treatment. Mike's parents divorced when he was 10 years old, and he was reared predominantly by his mother. At the time of the initial interview, Mike was a strong prospect to continue football in the pro ranks. Other than football, he did not mention alternative plans for his future.

DIAGNOSTIC SUMMARY

Mike's diagnostic picture contains several characteristics that, in combination, suggest significant current problems with alcohol (that appear to meet DSM-IV diagnostic criteria for alcohol abuse), possible problems with other drugs, and potential for more serious problems in the future. Considered chronologically, these characteristics are coming from a divorced family, having a brother and father with substance abuse problems, inconsistent academic performance, alcohol use or abuse and at minimum experimentation with other drugs during high school and college, alcohol-related legal incidents such as the DUI charges, and other behavioral incidents that may or may not be alcohol related, such as missed curfews, arguments with teammates, and problems with the coaching staff. This history, combined with Mike's anger and resentment regarding his referral for treatment, suggests that there may be reasons for concern, not only for his alcohol and drug use but also for his mental health.

CASE STUDY

Ed

Ed was a 41-year-old, self-referred professional golfer who came for counseling initially because of "problems in my marriage." Ed appeared anxious during the initial interview and indicated that he had been feeling depressed the last several months. He stated that his wife had been upset with him for a variety of reasons but mostly because she thought he was drinking too much and should get help. When asked about his drinking, Ed replied he drank every day (between one and two pints of vodka) and that his drinking began in the evening after he had either been practicing golf or playing in a tournament. However, after stating this, he indicated that frequently his drinking would start at the clubhouse following his golf round when he would "drink a few with the guys." He indicated that this pattern of drinking had begun when he started his professional golf career following college at the age of 22. He also indicated that the volume of alcohol he drank gradually increased over the years, and increased amounts of alcohol had been necessary to achieve the effect he desired. He stated that it had been more difficult for him to get up and going in the morning after an evening of drinking. On occasion he had taken a drink in the morning to steady his nerves.

Ed indicated that he attempted to quit drinking approximately five years ago and was successful in staying abstinent for six months. He returned to drinking after he had several poor tournaments and was having difficulty relaxing after playing. Ed denied other drug use besides alcohol and indicated that, although he often drove under the influence of alcohol, he had not experienced any legal consequences from drinking. He indicated that at times he had drunk too much at social occasions and had behaved foolishly and was embarrassed about it after he "sobered up the next day."

Ed described himself as a shy person and recalled that during adolescence he felt uncomfortable in social situations. He stated that playing golf had been a passion for him since his teenage years and he had felt most comfortable during that time on the golf course. He described his earliest experiences with alcohol during high school as being sporadic but also as enjoyable. He remembered his first use of alcohol at age 15 as exciting and relaxing at the same time. He stated that alcohol seemed to permit him to feel more comfortable around people and to open up emotionally and express his feelings. He felt people responded to him better after he had a few drinks. Although there was no history of alcohol and drug abuse in Ed's family, he reported that his mother experienced problems with depression and had taken medication at times for this problem.

Ed's performance on the golf tour had been inconsistent recently and he expressed concern that his marital problems had affected his performance. Although he seemed concerned about his drinking, he did not attribute his decline in performance to the effects of alcohol.

DIAGNOSTIC SUMMARY

Ed's description of his alcohol use and related problems suggest that his symptoms meet the *DSM-IV* diagnostic criteria for alcohol dependence. His reports suggest that he is experiencing tolerance to the effects of alcohol, he has experienced difficulties in controlling his drinking, alcohol use and recovery from its effects occupy a significant portion of each day, and his marital and possibly his occupational life have been negatively affected by his alcohol use. For Ed, alcohol became a coping mechanism for his social discomforts during adolescence. He apparently discovered the *social lubricant* qualities of alcohol during adolescence and gained social confidence from these effects. Another noteworthy issue for Ed is feeling depressed and the presence of depression in his immediate family. It is not uncommon for depression and alcohol abuse or dependence to co-occur and for each disorder to contribute to the other's development. His marital problems appear to be alcohol related as well and serve as a catalyst for him to seek treatment.

CASE STUDY

Ron

Ron was a 29-year-old pitcher who had been playing in the major leagues for the last five years. He had shown great promise in his first two years as a major leaguer, but in the last three years his performances had dropped off. This performance decline was threatening his position in the starting rotation and the coach was considering sending him back to the minor leagues. Ron's referral for assistance was prompted by the coach's concern regarding his performance and more recently by a DUI charge. During the intake interview, Ron was upset about his potential demotion to the minor leagues. He had difficulty sitting still during the interview and frequently expressed anger toward his coach. Ron explained his decline in performance as a "temporary situation." He indicated that he felt he had a strong spring training and he was ready to make a contribution to the team this year. When questioned about his recent DUI, Ron stated that he had a few too many at the bar that night with his friends, but he did not feel his driving was impaired (reports from the police department indicated Ron's BAC was .20). When questioned further about recent alcohol-related legal problems, Ron, after some hesitation, stated that he had three DUI charges in the last five years and lost his license for six months during that time. Ron reported that he drank daily, but he did not believe his consumption level to be different from his peers. Because he was a starting pitcher, his turn in the rotation occurred every four or five days, which meant that his time between starts was unstructured. He reported that his drink of choice was bourbon, which he usually consumed on the days he did not pitch. On these days, he would start drinking "around dinner time" and would typically stay up until midnight or one o'clock in the morning. He was not specific about the amount of alcohol he consumed in a drinking day, indicating that it was approximately six to eight drinks. He typically consumed these drinks in four to five hours. He estimated that he finished a quart of bourbon every three days. Although it was not a pattern, Ron stated that he would take a drink the following morning occasionally to "steady my nerves." Ron stated that he attempted to abstain from alcohol on those days he was scheduled to pitch and on the night before; however, he was not always successful in doing so. He also mentioned that his doctor had told him he had an ulcer and should discontinue drinking. Ron suggested that his abstinent days allowed his stomach to recover sufficiently.

Ron reported a family history of alcoholism; both his father and grandfather were heavy drinkers and died from alcohol-related health problems. He indicated that he started drinking beer in high school with his friends, mostly on weekends. He was drafted out of high school and began to drink hard liquor while he was in the minor leagues. Although he denied current use of other drugs, he indicated that during his stint in the minor leagues he tried marijuana and cocaine, but had not used either of these drugs since coming to the major leagues. Ron indicated that during his minor league days he drank daily and had begun to have occasional control problems on the mound. He said he had always prided himself on his stamina and his ability to prepare himself well to pitch in big games. He expressed some concern that recently he had lost both of these qualities. Although admitting to a concern over his loss of "competitive edge," Ron felt his coach was not being fair assuming that his performance would not be up to major league standards in the upcoming season.

DIAGNOSTIC SUMMARY

Ron's reported history is consistent with the *DSM-IV* diagnostic criteria for alcohol dependence. His drinking history suggests that he has become tolerant to the effects of alcohol and has experienced some withdrawal symptoms, particularly the day after heavy drinking the preceding evening. He has also experienced alcohol-related legal and possibly occupational consequences. He has attempted to regulate his drinking and confine it to the days he is not pitching; however, he has been inconsistent in his ability to do so. His strong positive family history for alcoholism suggests that he is at high risk for continued development of an alcohol problem. It is noteworthy that Ron's profession in some ways has contributed to the development of his alcohol problem. Because he had as many as five days off between pitching starts, he could drink heavily without any dramatic problems with his pitching performance. The limited structure supplied by his work as well as the travel demands, with accompanying stressors, likely facilitated the development of his alcohol problem.

Alcohol-Abusing Sport Professionals

The following case studies are examples of alcohol-related problems in coaches and a medical professional.

CASE STUDY

Scott

Scott was a 32-year-old assistant football coach at a major university. He assumed his current job three years ago with the hopes of developing his coaching skills to become more competitive for a head-coaching position. Scott was married four years ago and the couple had one child. During the first session, Scott indicated that he had come for help because he was having some difficulty adjusting to his new responsibilities as an assistant coach and to his role as husband and father. He indicated that he did his best to fulfill his responsibilities but was having difficulty maintaining himself. He stated that his wife felt he worked too much and that when he was home he was not talkative and often distant. Scott remarked that his job demanded a great deal of his energy, and during the season he was preoccupied as much as 12 to 15 hours a day with his coaching duties. This left little time to interact with his wife and child. Also, he had a difficult time relaxing when he got home and drinking alcohol (usually beer or vodka) enabled him to relax and get to sleep. He estimated that he typically drank six beers or a half pint of vodka during the evening before going to bed. His wife apparently had expressed concern about the amount and frequency of his drinking as well as the effects it had on his behavior. She reportedly had expressed anger that he withdrew from her and would not show affection either toward her or to their child. She had encouraged him to seek assistance about his drinking as well as other problems he was experiencing in adjusting to his coaching position and to their marriage.

Scott reported a normal childhood and adolescence and indicated that he started to drink while in college, usually beer with his football teammates. After college, his drinking was confined mostly to weekends, but since beginning his new coaching position and getting married, his drinking had become more common during the week. He reported no history of alcohol or mental health problems in his immediate family, and until the last two or three years he did not have concern about his alcohol consumption. Although he stated that he understood his drinking was upsetting his wife, he was unsure of the need to modify his drinking pattern.

DIAGNOSTIC SUMMARY

Scott's drinking is probably sufficient to meet the *DSM-IV* criteria for alcohol abuse, but his alcohol problem appears to be in its earliest stages. His recent marriage and job duties are significant stressors in his life, which he has had difficulty responding to effectively. Alcohol seems to be a coping mechanism enabling him to feel that he is managing his life roles adequately. Favorable prognostic signs for Scott are that he lacks a family history of alcoholism, he has some awareness that he is not adapting well to changing life circumstances, he seems to understand that alcohol is playing a less than helpful role in his ability to cope, and he has come to his first session as a self-referral even though he had encouragement from his wife.

CASE STUDY

Juanita

Juanita was a 50-year-old college tennis coach referred by a friend who was concerned about her drinking. Her friend indicated that Juanita had been a successful college tennis coach for the past 25 years, but recently she seemed to have lost her enthusiasm for coaching. Juanita came for the first session dressed in her warm-ups, explaining that she had a practice later that afternoon. She indicated that she was proud of her career as a college tennis coach and had enjoyed the many close relationships she had developed with players over the years. However, she stated that during the last year her work had become more arduous and she did not gain the same gratification she had earlier in her career. When questioned about what may have prompted her decreased satisfaction with her job a year ago, she indicated that it was then that she and her husband, David, started having problems in their marriage. Juanita felt that her husband started getting upset about the amount of time she was spending in her coaching duties. She stated that he continues to feel resentful about time she devotes to her work, which, in his perspective, prevents them from doing things as a couple. She also stated that when she and her husband spend time together they both tend to drink too much and often end up in a verbal confrontation over a variety of issues. She denied that these confrontations became physical at any time.

When questioned about her drinking history, Juanita indicated that she considered herself a social drinker most of the time except when she and David drank too much. She stated that most of her drinking occurred on the weekends and that she typically would consume three to four six packs of beer from Friday to Sunday. During the tennis season, however, she indicated that she did not drink at all on the day the team had a match. She did not feel her drinking had affected her ability to coach. Reports from the friend who referred Juanita suggested otherwise. Her friend indicated that players had complained to other coaches that Juanita had on occasion come to matches with alcohol on her breath.

Juanita started drinking in high school along with most of her close friends at the time. She drank sporadically in college but never suffered any serious consequences. She and David married when they were both 23 years old, and the couple had a child when they were 28. Juanita indicated that she lost her only child, Sarah, in an automobile accident when she was 10 years old. David was also seriously hurt in this accident, suffering a back injury, which continues to bother him today. Following the loss of her child, Juanita drank regularly because this seemed to be the "only thing I could do to handle the emotional pain." She felt that her relationship with David deteriorated after the loss of Sarah.

Juanita still has periods of depression that she attributes to not being able to emotionally overcome Sarah's death. She stated that her drinking usually increases during these periods of depression. During these times, which have lasted up to one month and have occurred as frequently as three times per year (one time being around the anniversary of Sarah's death), Juanita apparently isolates herself from other people and finds it difficult to carry out routine activities.

DIAGNOSTIC SUMMARY

Juanita's reported history suggests that she is experiencing significant life disturbances related to alcohol consumption and her difficulty adjusting to the death of her child. Her current drinking most likely meets the *DSM-IV* diagnostic criteria for alcohol abuse and may progress to alcohol dependence. In Juanita's case, it appears that her drinking initially became problematic following the death of her child. Subsequently, alcohol use became a way in which Juanita handled emotional difficulties within her marriage. It is likely that, because her husband was involved in the automobile accident that resulted in Sarah's death, there may be significant unresolved emotional conflicts within her marriage related to this accident. Juanita's use of alcohol is reason for concern, particularly within the context of her difficulty adjusting to Sarah's death. Her history suggests that she will need treatment attention devoted to several issues in addition to her alcohol abuse, including bereavement, marital conflict, and vocational issues.

CASE STUDY

Richard

Richard was a 45-year-old sports medicine physician referred by a colleague who had recently undergone treatment for a drug abuse problem. During the first session, Richard explained that he was only there to ask a few questions about his alcohol use but was not interested in any "long-term help." Richard discussed his alcohol use indicating that he found it helpful to relax with a drink when he returned home after work, between 7:00 and 8:00 p.m. He drank two or three drinks of bourbon and water before dinner, which he usually ate around 8:30 or 9:00 p.m. He would continue to drink until he went to bed between 11:00 and 11:30 p.m. because he felt it helped him sleep. He reported that he finished from one-half to one pint of bourbon per night. On the weekends, Richard reported that he usually drank more and his drinking would start before dinner at approximately 6:00 p.m. He estimated that he drank over a quart of bourbon on a typical weekend. Richard indicated that on Sunday evening he usually tried not to drink so he could be prepared for his next working week; he frequently was unable to refrain from drinking.

Richard indicated that he started drinking as a sophomore in high school and remembered that he enjoyed the first time he became drunk. During college he confined his alcohol use to the weekends with his fraternity brothers. He said that he primarily drank beer during college. Richard described his alcohol use during medical school as sporadic and fairly heavy following stressful periods in school, such as after important examinations. He also began to experiment with sedative-hypnotic drugs (e.g., Valium) to help him sleep and to calm his nerves when he felt anxious about upcoming examinations. He said at the time he did not feel particularly concerned about the drug use because his classmates were doing the same thing, and he considered his drug use to be temporary until he graduated from medical school. Indeed, he stopped using drugs after his residency when he went into private practice and joined a medical group specializing in sports medicine. However, his alcohol use began to increase during his early years in practice, and over the next 15 years gradually increased until it reached its present level during the last two years.

When questioned about why he was pursuing advice at this time, Richard indicated that he recently received a DUI when he attempted to drive home after having too much to drink at a party. He was embarrassed by the DUI and he didn't feel it would ever happen again. Part of the court requirements included him coming to see a professional to discuss his alcohol use. Richard stated that he did not see any reason to pursue further treatment and that he felt fully capable of handling his drinking. He stated that the DUI was the result of "poor judgment." He apparently was not required to report his DUI to the medical licensing board and was therefore not facing any sanctions on his license to practice medicine.

DIAGNOSTIC SUMMARY

Richard's alcohol consumption, although not causing any difficulties in his estimation (except perhaps the DUI), is probably causing him more problems than he is aware of, or admitting to, and will likely cause him significant problems in the future if not changed. His history suggests that he has developed tolerance to alcohol over the last 15 years, indicated by the increasing amounts of alcohol consumed daily. Furthermore, he has tried to limit his consumption unsuccessfully. Although he does not report alcohol-related psychosocial problems (e.g., family, legal, occupational) aside from the DUI, it is likely that some of these problems are occurring or will occur. Additional history-taking would determine if Richard's symptomatology meets *DSM-IV* diagnostic criteria for alcohol abuse or dependence. Given that he is a practicing physician, the welfare of his patients may depend on successful identification and appropriate intervention with his alcohol-related problems.

Also of concern in Richard's case is the pattern of his drug use during medical school. Apparently, he used sedative-hypnotics (drugs that have CNS-depressant effects similar to alcohol) to assist him in controlling anxiety and sleep. Although he terminated this drug use following medical school, his alcohol use continued and increased in the years following termination of drug use. Because alcohol and the sedative-hypnotic drugs have similar effects on the CNS, it is probable they are serving a similar function for Richard—they are a coping mechanism for dealing with anxiety and sleeplessness. A major drawback to their use as a coping mechanism for anxiety is that tolerance develops to their effects, which requires increased doses of the drug to yield the desired effects. With regard to sleeping difficulties, alcohol may be a temporary solution to induce sleep but, because of its rapid metabolism, is disruptive to normal sleep cycles. Therefore, it is likely that Richard's alcohol use will continue to escalate unless he develops alternative mechanisms to cope with anxiety and sleeplessness.

CASE STUDIES: SUMMARY OF ISSUES

These case studies exemplify many issues in assisting an individual with an alcohol-related problem. These issues are important, not only for the alcohol treatment professional, but also for any person referring an athlete or sport professional for treatment of an alcohol-related problem. Following is a discussion of these issues with references to the case studies. Where no reference is made, the issue applies to all the cases.

Continuum of Severity

The case studies exemplify the continuum of severity that underlies alcohol misuse (e.g., occasional alcohol-related problems without recurrent or significant adverse consequences), abuse, and dependence. Although factors of progression through this continuum are in debate, alcohol use of any kind carries with it the risk of misuse, abuse, and dependence. Certainly there are factors associated with increased risk for alcohol abuse and dependence, but the accuracy with which alcohol-related problems are predicted is limited. Therefore, helping professionals must know about the risks associated with alcohol use to communicate accurate information to athletes who may or may not be at risk for alcohol problems.

For the alcohol treatment professional, one of the first diagnostic decisions is to determine whether alcohol use constitutes misuse, abuse, or dependence. This gradation increases in seriousness and the outcome of this diagnostic decision suggests treatment differing in levels of intensity, setting, and length (see chapter 7). Those individuals who are misusing or abusing alcohol (Donna, Mike, Scott, Juanita, and perhaps Richard, although additional history-taking could verify that his symptomatology meets the DSM-IV criteria for alcohol dependence) often may be effectively treated in outpatient settings with varied treatment lengths and intensity depending on the number and severity of other presenting problems. Those who are alcohol dependent (Ed and Ron) frequently require time either in a hospital or a short-term residential facility. Some require extended outpatient treatment, which may last one year or longer.

Ambivalence About Change

People seek help for alcohol-related issues for various reasons, and frequently their help seeking is prompted by concern from others (e.g., spouse, coach, legal system). This is the case in varying degrees with all the examples. Because concerned others often initiate referral, it is not unusual for clients to be ambivalent about whether they have an alcohol problem, whether there is a real need for change, or whether they are capable of making changes if they determine that change is desirable. Most clients will need assistance examining these issues and will need guidance through various change strategies, depending on their situations (see chapter 6).

Confidentiality

Treatment for alcohol-related problems should occur in a highly confidential setting to allow for clients' maximum comfort in discussing sensitive issues without fear of this information being discussed with others outside the treatment context. Sensitive issues may include illegal activity, relationships with significant others, and potentially hurtful or embarrassing behavior engaged in while under the influence of alcohol or drugs. Effective treatment is based on a foundation of a mutually trusting relationship between the treatment professional and client, which starts with the assurance that information discussed will be kept confidential.

Diagnosing Coexisting Problems

Most alcohol abusers or dependents will have a variety of coexisting problems that require treatment concurrently with the treatment for their alcohol problem. These coexisting problems may range from medical and psychiatric problems to vocational and legal problems. These problems may predate and play some causative role in alcohol abuse (e.g., for Juanita the loss of her child appears to be associated with an increase in her drinking) or may be a consequence of the alcohol abuse (e.g., in Scott's case his drinking resulted in difficulties in his family relationships). The task incumbent on the treatment professional is to determine how these ancillary problems relate to the alcohol abuse and how to best treat them. Some problems may improve with the client's abstinence alone, but many will require additional therapeutic attention. For example, many alcohol abusers have experienced vocational problems related to inconsistent performance at work. Although their abstinence may lead to an improvement in their work performance, employers may mistrust the employee, which could undermine the development of an effective working relationship. The case examples of Ron and Juanita perhaps best exemplify this issue. Both will likely have to deal with regaining the trust and support of their employers during and after treatment of their alcohol-related problems. This task may involve various communications among the employer, client, and treatment provider, given appropriate consent from the client to the treatment provider to allow release of treatment-related information.

Sources of Diagnostic Information

Several important issues regarding the reliability of diagnostic information must be considered:

1. Individuals entering alcohol treatment will usually be ambivalent if not reluctant about or rejecting of some aspects of treatment, particularly if external pressures (e.g., the insistence of a spouse or employer) prompted their treatment. To the extent clients feel their freedom of choice is restricted, they may hesitate to share information, particularly when it pertains to their use of alcohol or other drugs. The skilled interviewer must be sensitive to this issue and design questions to allay fears and encourage candid answers from the client.

2. It is helpful to acquire information from multiple sources to provide a complete picture of the client's situation. Information sources may include family members, friends, employers, and workmates. Pursuing information from these multiple sources will not only provide a comprehensive picture of the individual but also will indicate the extent to which alcohol abuse has permeated various life spheres.

3. Comprehensive evaluation of alcohol abusers and dependents in treatment usually requires input from various professionals. Treatment programs may be staffed by professionals representing psychology, psychiatry, medicine, social work, nursing, counseling, vocational rehabilitation, clergy, and recreational or occupational therapy. The more serious the alcohol problem, the more likely it is that a multidisciplinary team will be required for successful treatment.

Validity of Self-Report Measures

The question often arises in alcohol treatment whether the self-report of alcohol and drug abusers can be depended on to be accurate, particularly regarding alcohol and drug use. It is usually the best policy to accept the validity of the individual's self-report unless there are persuasive reasons to believe otherwise. Potential reasons to suspect the alcohol abuser's self-report would be if the individual stands to lose something of value (e.g., a job, a significant relationship) if an accurate report is given or if the individual is being asked to account for alcohol use that happened in the distant past. Because alcohol has a direct negative effect on memory, the client, when asked to recount alcohol consumption happening several months ago, may simply not remember. Therefore, to the extent that the individual has no obvious reasons to distort the truth about alcohol use and is being asked to remember alcohol use within a reasonable time, self-report can be a reliable and valid indication of alcohol use.

Monitoring Alcohol and Drug Use

Many treatment programs use both breathalyzers and urine drug screens to monitor alcohol and drug use among clients. A breathalyzer can detect recent alcohol use; however, because alcohol is metabolized rapidly the breathalyzer has limited value in detecting alcohol. Therefore, it is important during the treatment process for the therapist and client to have an open and trusting relationship so the client will feel reassured that discussing episodes of alcohol use will lead to constructive problem solving rather than to rejection or chastisement. Treatment programs commonly use urine drug screens to monitor drug use by clients. Drugs are metabolized at various rates depending on the characteristics of the drug and the individual. Other drug use is often monitored even when the presenting problem is alcohol abuse, because abuse of other drugs is not uncommon among alcohol abusers. Urine drug screens are performed randomly so the client is unaware when a drug screen will be done, and the client receives feedback regarding the results of the drug screen. Negative results (indicating no drug use) can be an opportunity for praise and positive feedback regarding the client's treatment progress; feedback regarding positive results (indicating recent drug use) can be an opportunity to discuss relapse episodes and problem solve with the client to avoid similar episodes in the future.

Minimum Drinking Age

Although alcohol use is a well-accepted practice in the United States, for anyone under the age of 21 its use is illegal. Survey data indicate that experimentation with alcohol occurs with most young people during secondary school, and athletes are not exempt from this experimentation. However, it is important that professionals working with young athletes not condone its use in legally underage people. Therefore, if involved in counseling an athlete under age 21 (as with Donna), the health professional would be remiss if a discussion regarding illegality of alcohol use did not occur.

CONCLUSION

Alcohol abuse and dependence are a part of sport. Relevant literature suggests that athletes share risk factors for alcohol abuse and dependence with the general population; however, they also have risk factors related to their participation in sport. Similarly, sport professionals experience risk factors for alcohol abuse and dependence related to the demands of their professions.

If sport is to promote physical and mental health, it is incumbent upon sport professionals to be aware of circumstances that are antithetical to this goal. Alcohol abuse and dependence are two examples of conditions that restrict the potential of human beings. Knowledge of and therapeutic attitudes toward these conditions are the best ways for sport professionals to identify and intervene with athletes and colleagues who experience alcohol problems.

In the next chapter, we will explore ways in which sport professionals can take steps to prevent the occurrence of alcohol abuse and dependence.

5 SPORT-RELATED ALCOHOL ABUSE AND DEPENDENCE PREVENTION

Society knows what it wants to do about its alcohol problem but cannot find an effective way of doing it. It wishes to preserve the individual's freedom to drink for pleasure, but at the same time it seeks to curb the deviant behavior of those whose pleasure is drinking to excess. Where does the one stop and the other begin?

—R. Finn and J. Clancy

The best way to have a long-term impact on the incidence of alcohol abuse and dependence in the sport world is to develop well-conceived approaches to prevention. This chapter will explore how prevention has been handled on a societal level and will apply these principles to sport. We will start by examining the need for prevention, goals, and methods established nationally. The following sections discuss prevention approaches targeting individual and environmental factors associated with alcohol abuse and dependence. Where appropriate, I describe sport-related examples. The next section describes individuals within sport who may have significant impact on the effectiveness of prevention efforts. The chapter concludes with recommendations for developing successful prevention programs.

As in chapter 3, where much of the chapter is information on alcohol's effects on human functioning, this chapter devotes attention to prevention efforts for the general population. I have taken this approach because it is helpful to understand general prevention strategies to fully understand and appreciate sport-related prevention efforts.

NEED FOR PREVENTION

There is a tremendous need for prevention of alcohol and drug abuse in society. We recognize this need not only from a human and financial cost aspect but also from the awareness that prevention efforts can reduce alcohol- and drug-related costs to society. It has been estimated that in 1990 medical and other costs to society of alcohol abuse and dependence were $98.6 billion (Rice, 1993). Comparatively, tax revenues on alcohol were only $9.2 billion (U.S. Department of Commerce, 1992).

In response to the need for a comprehensive prevention effort, the Office of Substance Abuse Prevention (OSAP) was formed in 1988 to provide prevention and early intervention services for young people and, in particular, high-risk youth (Johnson, Amatetti, Funkhouser, & Johnson, 1988). In addition, in 1991 a statement of national health objectives entitled *Healthy People 2000* (USDHHS, 1991) incorporated a number of health status objectives involving alcohol and drug use, such as a reduction in deaths caused by alcohol-related motor vehicle crashes and a reduction in cirrhosis deaths. Also included were risk-reduction objectives, such as increasing the average age of first use of alcohol, reducing the proportion of young people who have used alcohol, and increasing the proportion of high school seniors perceiving social disapproval for heavy alcohol use.

Recent evidence suggests that efforts directed toward prevention are having a positive impact. There is an apparent overall reduction in alcohol use among youth during the last 15 years, a substantial decrease in alcohol-related traffic fatalities (particularly among drivers under age 18) partly attributed to changes in the minimum-drinking-age laws, and a general awareness of the economic savings to business and industry as a product of prevention efforts (USDHHS, 1993). Prevention efforts are receiving continued attention nationally as evidenced by a recent edition of *Alcohol, Health & Research World* ("Prevention of Alcohol-Related Problems," 1993), a publication of the Public Health Service, which was devoted exclusively to prevention of alcohol-related problems.

PREVENTION GOALS AND METHODS

In general, the goal of prevention efforts is to reduce the adverse effects of drinking, whether alcohol use is light, moderate, or heavy. Although past prevention approaches have focused on the negative consequences of alcohol abuse and alcoholism, more recent efforts have broadened the target to include social, legal, and economic factors that influence alcohol use. This change in focus has been prompted by an increased recognition that alcohol use pervades American society and, therefore, so do related problems. It also has been recognized that alcohol-related problems are not limited to the population of heavy drinkers. Light or moderate drinkers account for the majority of individuals experiencing problems with alcohol because they represent a much greater proportion of the population (Kreitman, 1986). Therefore, to be effective, we must target prevention at high-risk subgroups as well as the entire population of drinkers. To accommodate a broader focus, the public health model has been used to generate ideas for recent prevention efforts. This model emphasizes the interaction between host, agent (alcohol), and environment and suggests that we must not limit prevention of alcohol-related problems to the drinker (host) but must include attention to both host and environment (Wallack, 1983). Generally, strategies focusing on host factors relate to individual characteristics that may place a person at risk for alcohol problems (e.g., age, gender, and family history). Strategies devoted to environmental factors focus on characteristics of the environment that contribute to risk (e.g., accessibility of alcohol, alcohol-related laws).

Prevention efforts also have broadened with regard to objectives. Recent objectives have included decreasing negative consequences of acute and chronic drinking, such as traffic accidents and high-risk sexual activity associated with transmission of the HIV; preventing alcohol abuse and dependence; delaying the onset of alcohol use among youth; and promoting abstinence among individuals who should not drink (e.g., seriously head injured). It may be that rather than focusing on alcohol use, we should direct prevention efforts toward reducing risky behaviors generally, including excessive alcohol use, associated with adverse health consequences.

How do prevention efforts relate to the sport world? Perhaps a better question would be how do prevention efforts *not* relate to the sport world. Sport is an important institution in America, as well as other parts of the world, playing a major role in socialization. Only 3.7 percent of the U.S. population is unaffected by sport; in other words, these individuals do not participate in any fan or athletic event more than once a month. Teenagers in particular are avid sport participants, with approximately 66 percent of people 14 to 17 years of age participating in sport (Research & Forecasts, 1983). In addition, as indicated by Stuck (1990), youth involved in sport are like their nonathlete peers with regard to alcohol- and drug-related attitudes and behaviors. Therefore, in view of the broad overlap between alcohol use and sport participation, any alcohol abuse prevention efforts will most likely influence the sport world.

The following two sections of this chapter describe specific prevention strategies grouped as targeting individual and environmental factors contributing to alcohol use or abuse. In some cases both individual and environmental factors are targeted within a particular strategy and this will be noted. Further, individual and environmental approaches take three forms: (1) primary prevention, which typically seeks to prevent new cases of alcohol use or abuse, (2) secondary prevention, which seeks to identify early signs of alcohol-related problem behavior and induce the individual to either change alcohol use patterns or discontinue drinking, and (3) tertiary prevention, which seeks to terminate the compulsive use of alcohol and decrease associated negative effects through treatment and rehabilitation (Funkhouser & Denniston, 1992). We draw these distinctions in prevention strategies for definition purposes; there is often significant overlap between these categories. Indeed, successful prevention efforts typically incorporate all these prevention strategies.

PREVENTION DIRECTED TOWARD INDIVIDUAL FACTORS

Prevention efforts focusing on characteristics of individuals that place them at risk for alcohol abuse or dependence include education, screening, brief interventions, interventions with drinking drivers, employee assistance programs, and prevention with children of alcoholics.

Educational Approaches

We can divide educational approaches into programs based in and targeted for the community at large and programs designed for children, youth, and young adults in school.

Community Education Programs. Community education programs often use a variety of prevention strategies, including mass media campaigns, educational meetings with various citizen groups (PTA, employers), training in monitoring blood alcohol concentration (BAC), and discussion of alcohol policy in the media. Also included in this genre are grass roots programs such as Mothers Against Drunk Driving (MADD), Students Against Driving Drunk (SADD), and Remove Intoxicated Drivers (RID). Mass media campaigns alone do not effectively change health behaviors. However, these campaigns can increase awareness and provide a context for other prevention strategies to be effective (Funkhouser, Goplerud, & Bass, 1992). Of great importance to the success of these community education endeavors is the cooperation of community members and institutions in program planning.

School-Based Programs. School-based alcohol prevention programs are designed to delay the onset of drinking in youth. There is significant evidence, however, that alcohol is a *gateway* drug, meaning that its use often precedes and leads to use of other drugs (Kandel, Yamaguchi, & Chen, 1992). Therefore, comprehensive substance abuse prevention programs often target alcohol and drug use together.

School-based substance abuse prevention programs have incorporated curricula designed to prevent the onset of alcohol and drug use. In a recent review of this literature, Hansen (1992) found that broad-spectrum programs incorporating diverse prevention strategies and programs emphasizing on peer and other social pressures and on teaching students skills to resist these pressures (social influence programs) were most effective in preventing substance use. In a separate but related review of alcohol prevention programs, Hansen (1993) found that programs designed to change normative beliefs regarding alcohol were most successful in preventing alcohol use. These programs focused on correcting erroneous normative beliefs about alcohol by encouraging students to discuss and debate issues related to the appropriateness of alcohol and other drug use. Prentice and Miller (1993) found that perceived social norms play a significant role in the attitudes and behaviors of college students regarding alcohol use. In agreement with Hansen, these authors recommended that prevention programs seek to change perceived social norms about alcohol use by encouraging students to speak openly among their peers about their private attitudes regarding alcohol use.

Such social influence prevention programs are often based on social learning theory and frequently emphasize the role of peer influence in alcohol and drug use. Therefore, peer leaders participate in planning and implementing these programs with apparent success.

Although our knowledge about effective school-based substance abuse prevention programs is not complete, we can make several general conclusions. Effective programs are comprehensive in their scope, paying particular attention to the social influences that determine alcohol use. Although alcohol-related knowledge dissemination (a pervasive component in prevention programs) is not enough in itself for effective prevention, it remains an important component of prevention programs to increase perceived personal susceptibility to negative consequences of drinking (Hansen, 1992; Stainback & Rogers, 1983).

Prevention for Athletes. Although efforts continue in researching the most effective substance abuse prevention strategies, the literature has reported promising approaches with athletes using some of the described prevention methods. One example, described by Woolf (1986), is a comprehensive drug abuse prevention program targeted for high school athletes in the Forest Hills School District in Cincinnati, Ohio. Sponsored jointly by the National High School Athletic Coaches Association, the National

Football League, the National Football League Players Association, the International Association of Chiefs of Police, and the U.S. Drug Enforcement Administration, this program assists coaches in developing effective alcohol and drug abuse prevention activities with their high school athletes. Although the program has not been rigorously evaluated, it is a good example of how we can cooperate to involve many institutions and individuals, both at the national and local levels, to increase awareness of alcohol and drug use among athletes and counteract this use (see appendix B, Deighan et al., 1986, for more information).

Other prevention efforts with high school athletes have sought to instruct them regarding the dangers of drug use and to encourage their leadership in modeling appropriate health behaviors (Griffin & Newman, 1989; Oberman, 1989; Palmer, Davis, Sher, & Hicks, 1989). These programs typically have two major purposes: prevent alcohol and drug use problems among athletes, and provide these athletes with the tools to influence both their age peers and younger students in middle and elementary schools. These programs frequently do not include rigorous outcome evaluation; however, participants and school and community officials appear to receive them well.

Prevention programs at the college level are similar to high school programs in that they promote collegiate athletes as effective role models for their peers and for younger students. A *Drugs in Sport* educational program developed at the University of Kansas consisted of didactic experiences in a one-hour classroom credit course for athletes and a role-modeling activity in which athletes made presentations to school children regarding drug abuse prevention (Lowcock, Cook, & Tricker, 1992). Although they focused primarily on *performance-enhancing* drugs, they also devoted time to *recreational* drugs, including alcohol. The text for the course entitled *Athletes at Risk: Drugs and Sport* (Tricker & Cook, 1993) was edited by professors at the University of Kansas who originally designed the course. Although extensive evaluation is unavailable, the authors reported positive responses to the course from the student athletes participating, as well as from the local community. It was emphasized that the program's success depended on a "solid commitment from the athletic department to provide a legitimate educational experience for the athlete" (Lowcock, Cook, & Tricker, 1992, p. 10).

Another approach to prevention with college, high school, and middle school athletes and nonathlete students is based on developing life skills. The Life Development Intervention Program, developed by Danish and D'Augelli (1983), seeks to develop competence across various domains and tasks by teaching goal setting and attainment skills. This intervention program has been applied in various contexts and recently used in preventing alcohol and drug abuse (Danish, Petitpas, & Hale, 1990).

One example of an application of this life skills program is the Athletes Coaching Teens (ACT) program, which uses sport to motivate high-risk, inner-city adolescents to decrease health-compromising behaviors (e.g., alcohol and drug use, violent behavior, unsafe sexual practices) and increase their health-enhancing behaviors. As described by Danish et al. (1990), "the ACT program teaches students 'what to say yes to' as opposed to 'just saying no'" (p. 186). The ACT program was part of a three-year substance abuse prevention demonstration project funded by the Office for Substance Abuse Prevention (OSAP). It was a comprehensive program in that it included a collaboration between the Department of Psychology at the Virginia Commonwealth University (VCU) and the Richmond City Public Schools. It included not only VCU staff but also professional, college, and high school athletes in program implementation. Therefore, it influenced athletes from the professional ranks to middle school youth.

A second application of the life skills program described by Danish et al. (1990) was a 10-week course entitled Success 101 that assisted student athletes in the transition from high school to college. A related intent of the program was to prevent student athletes' involvement with substance use. Underlying the program was a primary assumption that student athletes face tremendous demands in the transition from high school to college athletics and that they need guidance in learning how to cope with the demands of academics and athletics. Coping effectively requires such skills as goal setting, time management, enhanced decision making, and relaxation. The product of successful coping for the student athlete is achievement, both academically and athletically, and an increase in self-confidence. Alternatively, unsuccessful coping could lead to substance use, lack of emotional control, poor concentration, and other counterproductive behaviors. The usefulness of these skills is not limited to athletics. These are skills that will determine achievement levels throughout life. The authors suggested that interventions such as ACT and Success 101 may increase the likelihood that the student athlete will successfully transfer these skills from the sport context to future endeavors. Sport participation therefore would become a vehicle for developing personal competence across settings.

Screening

Screening identifies individuals who are either currently experiencing an alcohol-related problem or are at risk for developing one (i.e., a secondary-prevention population). Screening activities also may be done in populations without suspected risk for alcohol-related problems. For example, Umbricht-Schneiter, Santora, and Moore (1991) screened patients admitted to an academic medical center and found that 22.4 percent of patients were positively screened for alcohol abuse, which was significantly higher than the percentage of patients (7.4 percent) identified as alcohol abusers on discharge diagnoses, thus suggesting a need for regular screening efforts. Although mass screening may be appropriate and effective in some settings, it is infrequently done for various reasons, including cost and confidentiality issues (USDHHS, 1993).

Given the established validity of screening secondary-prevention populations for alcohol-related problems, screening may be done through interviewing, instruments designed for screening purposes, laboratory tests, or a combination of these approaches (see review in USDHHS, 1993). Methods used for screening have included face-to-face interviews conducted by nonclinicians and clinicians, paper-and-pencil questionnaires, and self-guided computerized interviews. The validity of these methods is apparently similar, which argues for using paper-and-pencil and computerized methods for cost efficiency. Additional research is needed to develop valid screening instruments for subpopulations such as ethnic minorities, women, and older adults.

Although it is a common assumption that direct questions about alcohol consumption will not yield valid information because people tend to deny problems related to their alcohol use, recent reviews (e.g., Sobell & Sobell, 1990) suggest that self-reports of alcohol use are important sources of data. Skinner (1984) suggested that validity of self-reports of alcohol use rely on various factors, including recency of client alcohol consumption, client physical and mental stability, client and interviewer rapport, client awareness of corroborating alcohol-related lab tests or collateral reports, assurance of client confidentiality, and appropriate interviewer questions regarding alcohol consumption. Questions often focus on quantity and frequency of alcohol consumption. Although these questions may be phrased differently, use of specific methods has demonstrated positive effects on validity of self-reports. These methods include asking about specific amounts of alcohol rather than average amounts; defining the amount of alcohol in a single drink; asking about specific amounts of beer, wine, and spirits consumed; and inquiring about frequency, quantity, and heavy use in different questions (see review in USDHHS, 1993).

Though screening and identifying drinkers experiencing alcohol-related problems or those at risk for doing so is an important activity, the task is more difficult than identifying drinkers with severe problems. As depicted in figure 5.1, a variety of psychosocial and biomedical problems can relate to alcohol abuse in its early stages; however, these signs are more subtle and less consistent than symptoms that occur later in the progression of an alcohol problem (Skinner, 1986). In addition, drinkers are less likely to be forthcoming with information about potential alcohol-related problems earlier in the development of alcohol abuse. Consequently, screening and identification efforts must be proactive and occur in a variety of settings to be successful in identifying candidates for early intervention.

Screening Youthful Populations. Screening and identifying individuals with alcohol-related problems are pertinent to youthful populations as well. As discussed in chapter 2, most youth will begin experimenting with alcohol during adolescence and some will drink at a level that is reason for concern.

The task of identifying youth at risk for developing alcohol-related problems is aided by the fact that health-compromising behaviors frequently come in groups (Newcomb & Bentler, 1988). Alcohol and drug use are only one example of at-risk behavior. Other examples include unprotected sexual activity, delinquency, and dropping out of school (Dryfoos, 1990). It has been estimated that up to 50 percent of youth are at moderate to high risk for mental health problems based on exhibiting one or several of these at-risk behaviors. This high percentage of youth at risk for adverse health outcomes emphasizes the seriousness of the problem and the need for intervention to promote both physical and mental health among adolescents (Kazdin, 1993).

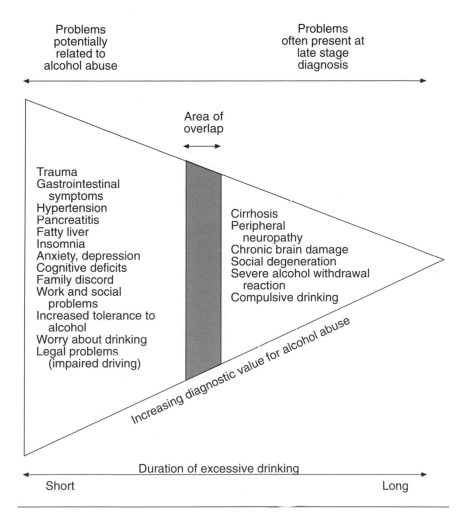

Figure 5.1 Disorders associated with the duration of excessive drinking. Disorders in the column on the left are potentially related to alcohol abuse. Disorders in the column on the right frequently are associated with late stage diagnosis. The area of overlap represents transition from potential early signs to more definitive diagnostic indicators of probable alcohol dependence. The triangle represents the increasing diagnostic value of symptoms as excessive drinking continues.

From "Early Intervention for Alcohol and Drug Problems: Core Issues for Medical Education" by H. A. Skinner, 1986, *Australian Drug and Alcohol Review,* 5, p. 71. Copyright 1986 by The Australian Medical and Professional Society of Alcohol and other Drugs. Published by Carfax, P.O. Box 25, Abingdon, Oxfordshire OX14 3UE, United Kingdom. Adapted with permission.

Brief Interventions

Once an alcohol-related problem has been identified, relatively brief interventions can effectively alter the course of harmful alcohol use (see reviews by Bien, Miller, & Tonigan, 1993; Institute of Medicine, 1990). Brief interventions vary in content and may include an assessment of an alcohol problem by a professional, feedback to the individual regarding drinking and its effects, behavior modification techniques and a self-help manual to assist the individual to change drinking behavior, and follow-up to monitor progress. General health care and alcohol treatment settings have used brief interventions successfully. It has been found in each of these settings that brief, well-constructed interventions can change drinking patterns and often are as effective as more extensive treatment (Bien et al., 1993). Chapter 6 includes a more detailed discussion of brief interventions and principles underlying the change process in problem drinkers.

Moderate Drinking. Recent reviews of the literature have suggested that moderate drinking, as opposed to abstinence, may be an appropriate goal for nondependent drinkers experiencing adverse effects of alcohol use (Marlatt, 1988; Miller & Hester, 1986a, 1986c). Factors that appear to predict positive outcome from moderation training include lower duration and severity of drinking-related symptoms and problems (Miller & Hester, 1986c). A method called Behavioral Self-Control Training (BSCT) has been most frequently used to teach moderate drinking skills (Miller, 1984). Table 5.1 lists the strategies typically included in BSCT. This and related methods have been used with DUI offenders and various self-referred adult populations with success in reducing alcohol consumption and alcohol-related problems. This strategy also has been used with young-adult and high-risk adolescent populations to reduce potential harm from alcohol use (Kivlahan, Marlatt, Fromme, Coppel, & Williams, 1990; Marlatt, Larimer, Baer, & Quigley, 1993). Although continued research is needed to identify the intensity and type of BSCT (e.g., therapist-conducted, provided by a self-help manual, or a combination of both) best for specific populations, this approach is promising as a prevention strategy. Perhaps we can most appropriately regard BSCT and related therapies as intermediate therapeutic steps between brief interventions and specialized alcohol treatment. Providing these therapies would require more professional time and expertise

TABLE 5.1

Frequently Used Strategies in Behavioral Self-Control Training

Setting specific limits and goals for drinking

Using biofeedback or a blood alcohol concentration (BAC) table or estimation rules to teach BAC discrimination

Self-monitoring of alcohol consumption

Slowing drinking through use of rate-control methods

Using operant principles including self-reinforcement and self-contracting

Identifying frequent antecedents or consequences that affect drinking behavior

Altering antecedent conditions through stimulus control and teaching new skills such as drink refusal

Learning behavioral alternatives to drinking

Data from *Seventh Special Report to the U.S. Congress on Alcohol and Health* (p. 247) by the U.S. Department of Health and Human Services, 1990, Rockville, MD: National Institute on Alcohol Abuse and Alcoholism.

than brief interventions but would be vastly less intensive than specialized treatment.

Intervening With Drinking Drivers

Another excellent area for preventing alcohol-related problems is identifying and intervening with drinking drivers. Both license sanctions and treatment interventions (e.g., group therapy, moderation training) have been instituted with DUI offenders in an attempt to decrease DUI rearrests, automobile accidents, and subsequent drinking. Success rates have varied with license sanctions and treatment-related interventions, and more research is needed to determine the deterrent effects of sanctions and the possible therapeutic effects of interventions so that both traffic safety and rehabilitative goals may be realized (see review in USDHHS, 1990).

Research that has focused on differentiating DUI offenders from other drivers suggests that those at risk for DUI may exhibit a constellation of high-risk behaviors, part of which is impaired driving (Jonah, 1990). Other high-risk behaviors include excessive alcohol consumption, drug use, unhealthy behavior, and illegal activity. Youthful drivers may be prone to exhibit a similar constellation of risk-taking behaviors, which includes high-risk driving and other health-risk behaviors, such as smoking, other drug use, and delinquency (see review in USDHHS, 1990).

Although our knowledge of the psychosocial characteristics of impaired driving has increased, use of this knowledge in early identification and intervention has been sparse, particularly for young drivers. Because impaired driving often appears as part of a larger constellation of health-risk behaviors, efforts may need to be directed toward modifying lifestyle generally. Because lifestyle changes become more difficult with increasing age, perhaps the greatest efforts should focus on early intervention. For example, educational activities on drinking, impaired driving, stress management, and risk taking should be conducted before adolescence (i.e., ages 12–13), when these problem behaviors tend to appear (Jonah, 1990). Also, efforts should be made to identify those individuals at high risk for impaired driving and intervene with either education-based programs or treatment programs along with license sanctions.

Employee Assistance Programs (EAPs)

We can potentially identify problem drinkers in the work setting and facilitate appropriate intervention. Workplace strategies for prevention of alcohol abuse have included three components: employer policies, employee education and awareness campaigns, and EAPs (Funkhouser, Goplerud, & Bass, 1992). Employer policies can communicate expectations about alcohol and drug use directly to employees as well as policies regarding drug testing. Employee education and awareness campaigns can publicize employer policies and reinforce societal messages about alcohol and other drug misuse that may have been communicated elsewhere. EAPs help identify employees experiencing problems with alcohol and drug use, as well as other life problem areas that may decrease job performance. By way of constructive confrontation, EAPs assist individuals in seeking help. Although basing intervention on job performance may be helpful with later stage alcohol problems, it is possible that linking EAPs with company health promotion activities will assist in identifying and intervening with alcohol abusers earlier (Reichman, Young, & Gracin, 1988).

EAPs have potential to reduce alcohol-related work performance decrements as well as the negative effects of alcohol abuse on the individual; however, more research is needed to determine under what conditions they can be most effective. For example, areas needing investigation include the relative effectiveness of using job performance criteria to identify alcohol-compromised employees, labor-union-based assistance programs, the EAP self-referral process and population, and the effects of incorporating intervention and assistance for alcohol problems within the context of a broader EAP model (Roman, 1988).

Prevention With Children of Alcoholics

Although most offspring of alcoholics do not develop problems with alcohol themselves, these individuals are at higher risk for alcoholism than the general population. Research is ongoing into the psychological, social, and biological markers that characterize children of alcoholics who are at greatest risk to become dependent on alcohol. Related research (Werner, 1986) indicated that, although most children of alcoholics (COA) function well and do not have serious problems, many of these children suffer serious coping problems by young adulthood. A recent review (National Institute on Alcohol Abuse and Alcoholism [NIAAA], 1990) indicated that COAs suffer higher incidences of cognitive deficits, psychological disorders, and behavioral problems than their peers who do not have an alcoholic parent (non-COA). It is not clear presently whether these problems are specific to COAs or whether they occur with equal frequency in other dysfunctional families. This information is necessary to construct suitable interventions and to justify committing health resources to implement screening and intervention programs for this at-risk population (Blane, 1988).

Though many studies suggest that differences exist between COAs and nonCOAs, methodological limitations of these studies, as well as an inadequate number of comprehensive studies, prevent conclusions about all COAs (NIAAA, 1990). At best, parental alcohol dependence should be regarded as a risk factor for alcohol use problems and other psychological and behavioral problems in their offspring and should serve as a basis for communicating this risk to COAs (Blane, 1988). Considering this risk factor, along with other relevant psychosocial factors, will allow each individual to make appropriate decisions about alcohol use.

PREVENTION DIRECTED TOWARD ENVIRONMENTAL FACTORS

Environmental factors play an important role in use and abuse of alcohol and serve as legitimate targets for prevention. A variety of environmental variables influence amount and frequency of alcohol consumed in a population as well as the occurrence of alcohol-related negative consequences. Examples of these variables include the availability of alcohol, advertising of alcoholic beverages and other ways the media portrays alcohol, legislative and policy factors potentially influencing drinking (e.g., minimal drinking age laws, drinking-and-driving laws), education and training programs for individuals who may intervene with alcohol users and potentially prevent negative consequences (e.g., servers of alcoholic beverages, health care professionals, adolescents who may prevent intoxicated peers from driving), and provision of transportation alternatives for drinkers (USDHHS, 1990).

Availability of Alcohol

A recent review (USDHHS, 1993) indicated that alcohol availability is linked to alcohol consumption and related problems. Alcohol availability is defined across several dimensions. These include physical availability (usually measured in terms of outlet density); economic availability (measured by price of alcoholic beverages and income of consumers); legal availability (affected by laws governing the sale of alcoholic beverages); and social and subjective availability (referring to the influence of lifestyle and routine activities on perceived availability of alcohol). These types of availability are important in determining alcohol consumption; however, we have yet to explore their importance in preventing alcohol-related problems.

Advertising of Alcoholic Beverages

There is continued interest in the effects of advertising alcoholic beverages on consumption rate. To date, reviews have differed in their conclusions regarding this relationship. A recent review by Smart (1988) concluded that (a) advertising bans have not shown significant influences on alcohol sales, (b) no consistent relationship has been demonstrated between alcohol sales and restrictions or funds spent on advertising, and (c) experimental studies have inconsistent results but the best designed studies show no impact of advertising on alcohol consumption. Conversely, Atkin (1987) concluded that advertising may play a significant contributing role in creating or reinforcing maladaptive patterns of alcohol use.

The concern over the influence of advertising on alcohol consumption is most pronounced in college student populations. College students have high rates of heavy alcohol consumption compared with their noncollege age mates and experience significant related, negative consequences, such as academic problems, trauma, date rape, and vandalism (Ryan & Mosher, 1991). These alcohol-related problems among college students prompted college and university presidents to declare alcohol the number one health problem on university campuses (from a national survey of college and university presidents cited in Ryan & Mosher, 1991, p. i). A recent progress report on alcohol industry marketing on college campuses (Ryan & Mosher, 1991) suggested that despite a moderation of aggressive marketing on campus, continued efforts are needed to restrict access of alcohol advertisers in school newspapers, at stadiums, and at other school-related events. In addition, the report recommended that colleges and universities develop comprehensive alcohol polices, including student participation, with the intent of promoting a safe and healthy campus environment.

Legislation and Policy

Another environmental prevention strategy is to use legislation or policies either to influence alcohol consumption levels or to prevent adverse consequences of alcohol consumption. Laws and policies communicate society's attitudes regarding alcohol use and provide support for other preventive efforts, such as education (Funkhouser, Goplerud, & Bass, 1992). Recent examples of legislation intended to prevent alcohol and drug abuse are the congressional passage of the Drug-Free Work Place Act (1988) and the Drug-Free Schools and Communities Act (1986). These legislative acts have focused attention on the problems surrounding alcohol and drug use in the work setting, as well as by youth, which have threatened the safety of employees and students and the organizational missions of businesses and schools. Although it is still early to evaluate the effectiveness of these legislative acts, it appears that they have mobilized preventive efforts nationwide, both in the public and private sectors.

Other legislative measures that have shown desirable effects in preventing alcohol-related problems include the section entitled "National Minimum Drinking Age" found in Title 23 of the U.S. Code Annotated at section 158 ("23 USCA," 1990) which encouraged all states to raise the minimum legal drinking age to 21; restrictions on the number and types of outlets that may sell alcoholic beverages and the hours they may operate; drinking-and-driving laws that have combined license suspension and educational programs designed to reduce the incidence of drinking and driving; and the so-called dram shop or liquor liability laws, which hold the server of alcoholic beverages liable for injury or damage caused by an individual who was served alcohol inappropriately (e.g., if intoxicated or under age). These legislative approaches to prevention have demonstrated some positive effects on alcohol consumption and related problems; however, additional evaluation is needed to refine these approaches so they yield more benefits. A review of the literature on these prevention measures is contained in the *Seventh and Eighth Special Reports to the U.S. Congress on Alcohol and Health* (USDHHS, 1990, 1993).

Policies at the organizational level also may have influence on alcohol and drug use and consequences. Most sport leagues or organizations (amateur and professional) have policies and programs to discourage alcohol and drug abuse and assist those athletes needing treatment (see Wadler & Hainline, 1989, for examples). Similar policies and programs are found at the collegiate level (reference to be obtained). Too often, however, these policies focus primarily on handling drug abuse, with scarce or no mention of alcohol use by athletes. For example, in a survey of 272 women's sports programs in the NCAA, Young and Young (1989) found that 68 percent of Division I and 53 percent of Division III programs had no departmental policy addressing alcohol use by student athletes. Lack of policies is bypassing an excellent opportunity to communicate expectations regarding alcohol use and possibly to prevent alcohol-related problems among athletes.

Potential Intervention Agents

Another potentially fruitful area for prevention by changing environmental risk is to educate those individuals who may be able to regulate access to alcohol or to identify individuals who may cause themselves or others harm because of alcohol use. Examples of these individuals are servers of alcoholic beverages, health professionals, and adolescents who may be able to intervene with friends intending to drive while intoxicated.

Servers. A review by McKnight (1993) indicated that training servers of alcoholic beverages in serving practices can be effective in reducing how fast and how much customers drink. However, he emphasized that achieving true responsible alcohol service relies heavily on public awareness of the problem of irresponsible alcohol use, community leadership in recognizing the need for responsible alcohol service, enforcement of alcohol control laws, management support of responsible alcohol service policies, and finally, effective server training programs that translate policies into action. An excellent example of a sport-related, community-based program that emphasizes server training is the Techniques for Effective Alcohol Management (TEAM) project. Briefly described in chapter 2, this project is a collaborative effort between public and private agencies and is geared for creating a more enjoyable game atmosphere at sporting events by decreasing drug- and alcohol-related incidents (Impellizzeri, 1988). Part of the TEAM approach is to instruct servers of alcoholic beverages and other employees at sport events to recognize symptoms of alcohol-related impairment in customers and take appropriate actions to prevent problems and ensure the safety of the drinker and others. Although a rigorous evaluation of the TEAM project has not been instituted, this comprehensive approach to prevention warrants further investigation.

Health Professionals. Health professionals are often in an excellent position to identify patients at high risk for health problems from their drinking and to facilitate changes in their drinking behavior. Recent prevalence studies have indicated that incidence of alcohol abuse and dependence in ambulatory, primary care (Cherpitel, 1991) and in hospitalized patients (Umbricht-Schneiter, Santora, & Moore, 1991) was 22 percent. A previous review of prevalence studies of alcoholism in hospital settings (Lewis & Gordon, 1983) suggested that prevalence may be as high as 55 percent in some hospitals. Unfortunately, however, many physicians apparently do not feel competent to treat or feel ambivalent about treating patients with alcohol and drug problems (Kennedy as cited in Funkhouser, Goplerud, & Bass,

1992). This is probably because most physicians do not receive adequate attention in their medical training to assess and treat substance abusers (Lewis, Niven, Czechowicz, & Trumble, 1987) and therefore do not feel comfortable in treating this population. A recent study by Roche and Richard (1991) indicated that general practice physicians often have a willingness to intervene with substance-abusing patients but may lack the requisite skills to do so effectively. Although interest has been stimulated in teaching substance abuse assessment and intervention strategies to health care students and practicing professionals (Dube, Goldstein, Lewis, Cyr, & Zwick, 1989; Lewis et al., 1987), much progress is needed in this area, not only for physicians but also for allied health care professionals (psychologists, social workers, nurses, etc.). As we will discuss in chapter 6, brief interventions with problem drinkers by health professionals have demonstrated effectiveness in reducing subsequent alcohol consumption.

Teenagers. Teenagers who are often placed in a position of riding with intoxicated peers may, if properly prepared, be able to prevent their peers from driving while under the influence of alcohol. A recent study suggested that adolescents may want to intervene with intoxicated friends but are not able to accurately judge their friends' incapacitation and may not be sufficiently skilled in intervening without negative confrontations (Turrisi, Jaccard, Kelly, & O'Malley, 1993). These results suggest that educational efforts be directed toward teaching adolescents the necessary skills to both recognize and intervene with intoxicated peers before they attempt to drive.

Transportation Alternatives

Another promising prevention strategy for reducing alcohol-related crashes is providing transportation alternatives to intoxicated drivers and their passengers. Transportation alternatives usually take the form of designated driver and ride service programs. Designated drivers are those individuals who are willing to remain sober and drive others in their group who are intoxicated. This strategy is most often used informally by groups of drinkers; however, some bars and restaurants have established formal designated driver programs (Apsler as cited in USDHHS, 1990). Ride service programs, on the other hand, are more formally organized and typically are sponsored by various organizations such as cab and bus companies, hospitals, charitable organizations, and police departments (Harding, Apsler, & Gold-fein, 1988). These programs provide intoxicated drivers alternative transportation. Though both designated driver and ride service programs are promising for preventing alcohol-related accidents, neither have been rigorously evaluated.

PREVENTION AGENTS IN SPORT

With a plethora of prevention strategies available to reduce the negative impact of alcohol use and abuse, who in the sport world shall be responsible for implementing the strategics? The short answer to that question is everyone. Prevention agents may include school and sport administrators and other school and community leaders, coaches, health professionals (e.g., psychologists, physicians, athletic trainers, physical therapists, nurses, counselors), athletes, organizations, and parents. Although none of these groups can take full responsibility for implementing prevention strategies, working together they can make a comprehensive network of prevention efforts that is most likely to succeed in reducing alcohol-related problems.

Administrators and Other Leaders

Being in a position to exercise influence on policy making and implementation, school, university, and other organizational administrators and leaders may set the tone for prevention efforts early. The most effective policies for alcohol and drug use and abuse prevention are products of collaborative discussion and decision making between affected parties, which may include organizational managers, coaches, teachers, parents, and appropriate community leaders. In the case of professional sport, the participants in this policy-making process might change but tasks remain essentially the same. An excellent example of this conjoint effort among secondary school athletes and fine arts participants is the experience of the Minnesota State High School League, which formulated a statewide policy for all school members (Svendsen, Griffin, & McIntyre, 1984). A primary reason for the successful development and implementation of these policies statewide was that school administrators made great efforts to include a variety of participants in an ad hoc committee charged with developing the policies. Committee members included school administrators, coaches, school board members, students, community agencies, and a state legislator. In addition, testimony was sought from school officials, coaches, law enforcement officials, clergy, parents, students, and community service agencies that was influential in the committee's development of a philosophy to underlie policy making.

Although the experience of the Minnesota State High School League was a successful one, there also are examples of unsuccessful attempts at policy formulation that we can learn from. For example, Lockwood and Saunders (1993) reported an unsuccessful attempt to formulate a comprehensive policy on alcohol and drug use at a university in Australia. They conjectured that the experience was unsuccessful because of poor processes (e.g., lack of effective consultation, suspicions about origins of the policy) underlying policy formulation. Further, they indicated that the major lessons learned were that policy formulation, presentation, and negotiation are tasks requiring a range of skills, including listening to criticism, consulting effectively, and instituting change slowly.

Coaches

Coaches are an excellent and largely untapped resource for alcohol-related problem prevention. They potentially may be the most important agents in preventing alcohol use and abuse on sport teams because of the tremendous influence they have on their players (Anshel, 1991). A survey by the National Youth Sports Coaches Association in 1989 (cited in Bakker, 1992) suggested that many athletes would look to their coach as a role model and as an alcohol and drug educator. Although there is some question about the extent to which coaches should become involved in regulating athletes' behaviors, such as alcohol and drug use, away from the sport context (Anshel, 1991), their potential value in prevention efforts must not be ignored.

To be effective as prevention agents, coaches must educate themselves about the problem of alcohol use and abuse among athletes, become aware of what preventive role they might play, and be comfortable carrying out activities within this role. Such activities may include stimulating a dialogue with athletes on alcohol and drug use, becoming knowledgeable of signs and symptoms of alcohol and drug abuse, and enforcing all training rules consistently with their athletes (Drug Enforcement Administration, 1986). Depending on their level of expertise and comfort, coaches can become involved in a variety of additional prevention efforts, as suggested by Anshel (1991), focusing on cognitive and behavioral approaches that may decrease the probability of alcohol and drug use. For example, cognitive approaches might include showing concern for the athletes' well-being as it pertains to alcohol and drug use, setting limits and controls on behavior, and teaching effective coping skills. Examples of behavioral strategies include helping the athlete avoid boredom by planning stimulating practices and scheduling recreational programs that are unrelated to the sport; taking an interest in the athlete's life situation outside of sport; and modeling appropriate and desired behavior. A recent evaluation of a chemical health education program for high school athletic coaches (Corcoran & Feltz, 1993) indicated that educational efforts can increase coaches' knowledge of chemical health issues and increase their confidence in applying that knowledge to their specific coaching situations.

Health Professionals

Health professionals also may provide valuable prevention services directly and indirectly. If sufficiently knowledgeable about signs and symptoms of alcohol abuse, health professionals treating athletes can identify alcohol abuse problems, perhaps in their early stages, and either intervene or refer the athlete for assistance. Indirectly, health professionals can help educate other prevention agents regarding health consequences of alcohol use and abuse, signs of alcohol abuse, and methods to facilitate early intervention and treatment. Before embarking on any of these endeavors, however, the health professional needs appropriate training and experience so their assistance can be effective rather than counterproductive. Because most health professionals lack training in alcohol and drug abuse prevention and treatment, additional education may be required for them to successfully carry out this role.

Athletes

Athletes themselves also may play a valuable role in prevention. If we are to minimize alcohol abuse problems in the sport world, athletes must not only take actions to reduce their own risk of alcohol abuse but also take responsibility for assisting their peers to do the same. One example of athletes taking action to help athletes is the United States Athletes Association (USAA), which is a member-supported network of chapters based in junior and senior high schools, colleges, and communities across the United States (Eller, 1988). Its primary, prevention-oriented mission is to prepare student athletes for the stresses of athletic competition and other endeavors after athletics by improving communication, human relations, and problem-solving skills.

ALCOHOL ABUSE PREVENTION PROGRAMS: COMPONENTS OF SUCCESS

As we have seen in this chapter, prevention programs have sought to decrease alcohol abuse and its related problems with varying levels of success. Based on a review of the general literature on alcohol abuse prevention as well as literature specific to prevention in sport, recommendations can be made to enhance the likelihood of success. Following, we will discuss these recommendations along with brief comments.

1. Prevention programs must accurately assess the needs of the population they will serve, potential resources available to meet the need, and the desired outcomes of prevention efforts. Unfortunately, most prevention programs have not taken this important step of assessment and identification of desired outcomes, and therefore are reaction based and lack direction, accountability, and measurement of outcome (Wilmes, 1993). Although reaction-based prevention programs do have strengths, they will not be able to provide the consistent effort needed for a sustained effect on alcohol abuse. A recent publication by the Substance Abuse and Mental Health Services Administration (Kimmel, 1993) may be a helpful guide to those charged with assessing needs in developing prevention programs.

2. The program must develop a clear philosophy of prevention along with supportive policies, goals, objectives, and methods (action plan) to reach the goals. We can best accomplish this process by including a variety of relevant community, professional, organizational, and athlete representatives to reach consensus of philosophy and direction for the program. Because alcohol use pervades our society and involves a number of its institutions, representatives on this planning body should include legal and law enforcement officials, clergy, health professionals, school officials, and parents and students (if policy development is for a school setting). To be effective, prevention programs must be comprehensive and coordinated in their ap-

proach to the problem of alcohol and other drug abuse (Cook & Roehl, 1993; Johnson et al., 1990; Substance Abuse and Mental Health Services Administration, 1992). Alcohol-related policies in schools, particularly in sport-related situations, have been challenged in the courts ("Arkansas—Court Finds,"1989; "Ohio—Wrestling After,"1991; Wong, 1988) and therefore must be carefully constructed to withstand legal scrutiny. A recent publication by Lewis, James, Hastings, and Ford (1992) gives practical guidelines for administrators and educators in constructing effective and legally defensible alcohol and drug policies. Public and private recreational facilities also are vulnerable to litigation regarding alcohol-related liability and must take similar precautions in instituting policies to prevent injury and property damage from alcohol abuse (Kozlowski, 1989; Pollard, Abraham, & Douglas, 1989).

3. Prevention programs should address both individual and environmental factors related to alcohol use as much as possible, and prevention strategies should be complementary. Prevention programs must acknowledge that alcohol use and abuse is a product not only of individual susceptibilities but also of environmental factors, which may increase or decrease the probability of alcohol use or abuse. Although focusing on many levels in prevention efforts is a challenging proposition, it is only through comprehensive effort that we will make enduring changes in alcohol abuse and related problems (Mason, Lusk, & Gintzler, 1992).

4. Prevention policies should be proactive; they should seek to either prevent alcohol-related problems from occurring or to intervene with them as early as possible in their development. In addition, prevention efforts should reinforce the positive behaviors of the majority of athletes who do not exhibit alcohol-related problems.

5. Programs should emphasize preventive and habilitative rather than punitive measures. Although punitive measures are necessary in some instances, it is more constructive to assist athletes in developing life skills that enable them to successfully negotiate their lives without abusing alcohol. This approach has been applied in sport-related settings with success and promise for the future (Danish, Petitpas, & Hale, 1990).

6. When punitive measures (e.g., suspension from athletic participation) are needed, they should be clearly communicated beforehand, consistently and equitably administered, and given

123

in conjunction with opportunities for corrective actions. When applied in this fashion, punitive measures have a role in prevention but certainly should not be relied on exclusively.

7. Program administrators should learn from the successes and failures of prevention programs already in existence. Although prevention is in its infancy, there are examples of prevention programs at the secondary-school, collegiate, and professional athlete levels that have achieved various successes (see appendix B containing resource information for prevention programs). Embrace the lessons from these programs and use them to forge more successful programs in the future.

8. Evaluation should be part of the prevention plan. A common problem identified in many alcohol and drug prevention programs is lack of evaluation (U.S. General Accounting Office, 1992). Too often evaluation is an afterthought when it should be a part of the initial plan for prevention. It is only through effective evaluation that program implementation can be monitored and progress measured toward identified outcome goals.

CONCLUSION

Prevention of alcohol abuse and dependence in the general population as well as in sport is a daunting responsibility. Effective prevention requires an understanding of the significant toll our society pays (both in human and economic loss) for the consequences of alcohol abuse and dependence. We must undertake the task of developing goals and methods for prevention with an appreciation that alcohol-related problems are diverse and affect a broad sector of the population. We must take a similar approach for prevention within sport because athletes are representative of the general population, including their alcohol use. Therefore, this chapter was purposely comprehensive in covering prevention approaches.

Prevention agents within sport must come from a variety of sources. Indeed, the probability of success in preventing alcohol abuse and dependence among athletes and sport professionals grows with the increasing breadth of participation among prevention agents discussed in this chapter. Furthermore, prevention must be ongoing. Alcohol use and abuse will always exist at some level within our society (if history is any indication), therefore requiring that prevention skills be among the armamentarium of effective helping professionals in sport. In the next chapter, we will explore ways that helping professionals can intervene with problem drinkers to prevent continued and more serious consequences of alcohol abuse from occurring.

6 HELPING THE PROBLEM DRINKER TO CHANGE

Nothing so needs reforming as other people's habits.

—Mark Twain

Assisting problem drinkers to change their behavior can be a challenging task for the helping professional. Fortunately, recent research on the process by which many individuals change addictive behaviors has provided useful guidelines. This chapter begins with a discussion of the natural history of alcohol dependence and the challenges faced in recovery. The majority of the chapter reviews stages that problem drinkers negotiate during recovery and ways that helping professionals may facilitate progression through these stages. The chapter concludes with a case study of an athlete with alcohol-related problems. The case study demonstrates interview strategies helping professionals can use to stimulate the change process.

NATURAL HISTORY OF ALCOHOL DEPENDENCE

In the United States, most people will have some experience with alcohol during adolescence and for many individuals this will be a time of repeated experimentation with drinking. For the majority of the population (85 percent to 90 percent of adults), drinking will be an activity done in moderation or not at all and will not pose significant health or social problems. For a subset of individuals, however, the initiation of drinking will lead to development of problem drinking, which may include alcohol abuse and dependence. This level of drinking is associated with various medical, social, legal, and psychological problems.

As movement occurs from initial alcohol use, to heavy social drinking, to alcohol abuse, and eventually to alcohol dependence, drinking becomes a well-established behavioral response. In many ways it becomes a coping mechanism to alleviate stressors, which may emanate from the environment, from the individual, and from the addiction process itself. Though some individuals may develop alcohol dependence over several years, for most individuals the process will take much longer. In a prospective study of American males, for example, Vaillant (1983) found that alcohol dependence took from 5 to 30 years to develop.

For those individuals who develop alcohol dependence, the process of recovery may be challenging. Although some alcoholics terminate their drinking without treatment (Tuchfeld, 1981), many individuals require intervention to assist them in recovery, whether it be formal treatment or attendance at a self-help group. Regardless of how an alcoholic initially recovers, the outcome for most individuals is relapse to alcohol use. Indeed, high relapse rates are common across all addictions, usually occurring within the first three months following treatment (Hunt, Barnett, & Branch, 1971). This treatment outcome data may invite pessimism; however, it has been suggested that recovery from alcohol dependence is a highly individual process marked by variations in use and abuse of alcohol (Armor, Polich, & Stambul, 1978). Distinctions need to be drawn between a lapse, or slip, which is a temporary return to alcohol use, and a relapse, which is a return to an addictive pattern of drinking (Brownell, Marlatt, Lichtenstein, & Wilson, 1986).

The remaining sections of this chapter will examine circumstances associated with successful recovery from alcohol-related problems and describe ways that helping professionals can facilitate this process.

CHANGING PROBLEM DRINKING: STAGES AND PROCESSES

Why and how do alcohol abusers and dependents change their addictive behaviors? As noted previously, successful change occurs both within and outside of treatment. In summarizing the results of his prospective study of alcoholics, Vaillant (1983) suggested that "alcoholics recover not because we treat them but because they heal themselves" (p. 314). He further suggested that this apparent reality should not negate the efforts of treatment personnel but should "redirect therapeutic attention toward the individual's own powers of resistance" (p. 315). Vaillant's line of reasoning perhaps is reflected in recent theories seeking to account for changes that individuals make in their addictive behavior. For instance, Prochaska, DiClemente, and Norcross (1992) have explored how addicted individuals change their behaviors. They have proposed an influential theoretical model suggesting that change occurs in stages that may take place within or independent from a treatment context. These stages include precontemplation, contemplation, preparation, action, and maintenance.

- *Precontemplation* is the stage in which there is no intention to change behavior in the immediate future. Most individuals are unaware or underaware of their problems at this stage and therefore are resistant to recognizing or modifying a problem. As described by G.K. Chesterton, "It isn't that they can't see the solution. It is that they can't see the problem" (cited in Prochaska et al., 1992, p. 1103).

- *Contemplation* is characterized by the individual being aware that there is a problem and thinking seriously about changing, but not being ready to commit to action. An important activity during the contemplation stage is the individual considering the advantages and disadvantages of the problem and the potential solutions to the problem.
- *Preparation* is typified by the individual intending to make changes, and perhaps beginning to move in that direction, but not yet having reached the point of sufficient action to terminate the problem. In the case of problem drinking, the individual may have made changes in drinking (e.g., reduced frequency and amount) but not have been able to reach criterion for effective action, such as abstinence from alcohol abuse.
- *Action* is the stage in which an individual takes direct action to overcome a problem. During this stage, the individual makes substantial overt efforts to change a problem behavior. For the problem drinker, this action may take the form of treatment, attendance at self-help groups such as Alcoholics Anonymous, or individual efforts to discontinue or moderate drinking.
- *Maintenance* is determined by the individual's efforts to prevent relapse and solidify behavior changes that have been made in the action stage.

As suggested by figure 6.1, progression through the stages is not linear, but is characterized by a relapsing and recycling process that individuals undergo while attempting to change addictive behaviors (what Prochaska et al., 1992, refer to as a spiral model of the stages of change). It appears that most relapsers recycle to the contemplation or preparation stages, potentially learn from their mistakes, and consider different strategies for the next action attempt. Therefore, cumulative effects of change attempts may be realized whereby the number of successful changers in a group increases gradually over time.

Prochaska et al. (1992) also proposed that during each stage of change specific processes occur that enable the individual to negotiate that stage. They described these change processes as

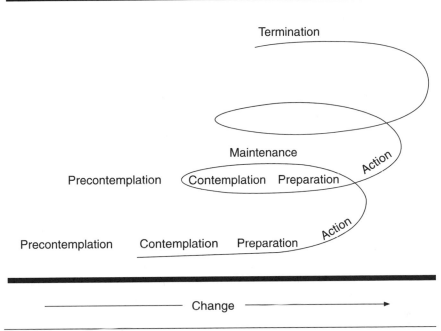

Figure 6.1 A spiral model of the stages of change.

From "In Search of How People Change: Applications to Addictive Behaviors" by J. O. Prochaska, C. C. DiClemente, and J. C. Norcross, 1992, *American Psychologist, 47,* p. 1104. Copyright ©1992 by the American Psychological Association. Adapted with permission.

"covert and overt activities and experiences that individuals engage in when they attempt to modify problem behaviors" (p. 1107). Examples of processes that individuals frequently use to change addictive behaviors are consciousness raising, self-liberation, and helping relationships. Consciousness raising refers to learning more about the problem and how one is reacting to it; self-liberation involves choosing and committing to an action and believing in one's ability to change; and helping relationships is being open and trusting about the problem with someone who cares. Various strategies can stimulate each of these processes, which an individual could use in therapy or without professional intervention by embarking on self-change.

The stage model of change has several important implications for how problem drinkers can make changes and how potential

131

helping agents can facilitate that process (Prochaska et al., 1992). The model stresses the following:

1. Assess the individual's readiness for change and design interventions to stimulate the processes the individual needs to successfully negotiate each stage of change.

2. Efficient change depends on applying the correct processes at the appropriate stage. If processes and stages are mismatched then change becomes more difficult. For instance, if interventions focus on the individual taking specific actions to change the addictive behavior (action stage) before the individual has reached sufficient awareness of the pros and cons of the problem and its potential solution (tasks associated with the contemplation stage), then the interventions and stage are mismatched and treatment outcome will likely be poor.

3. Most individuals seeking to change an addictive behavior will cycle through the stages many times before successfully accomplishing long-term maintenance. To expect the problem drinker to progress linearly through the stages and maintain abstinence, particularly after initial efforts, is to invite disappointment.

FACILITATING CHANGE IN PROBLEM DRINKERS

A recent national survey of prevalence and service use rates of mental and addictive disorders in the U.S. population during 1 year found that only 22 percent of alcoholics used any mental or addictive treatment services (Regier et al., 1993). In addition, most problem drinkers do not seek treatment (e.g., ratios of untreated to treated alcoholics range from 3:1 to 13:1; Sobell, Sobell, & Toneatto as cited in Sobell, Sobell, Toneatto, & Leo, 1993), and they typically do not discuss their drinking with health professionals until late in the course of the drinking problem after significant social impairment and pathological use of alcohol have occurred (Bucholz, Homan, & Helzer, 1992). However, it also has been found recently that the prevalence of natural recoveries from alcohol problems, (i.e., those occurring without treatment) may be greater than previously thought. For instance, Sobell et al. (1993) cited previous work by the Sobells that reported results from a Canadian national survey showing that of alcohol abusers who were recovered for a year or more, 82 percent reported recovering without treatment. In their recent study of individuals who resolved an alcohol problem without treatment, Sobell et al. (1993) indicated that over half progressed through a cognitive evaluation or appraisal of the pros and cons of drinking that contributed to their recovery. This cognitive appraisal process also has occurred in treated alcohol abusers (Amodeo & Kurtz, 1990).

Given these facts, how can helping professionals assist problem drinkers to make adaptive changes to their drinking behavior? Helping professionals may be most effective by stimulating the drinker's natural recovery capabilities, including cognitive evaluation of the pros and cons of drinking, a process that may or may not be underway.

Brief Interventions

A recent review by Bien, Miller, and Tonigan (1993) indicated that relatively brief interventions with alcohol abusers, which focus on this cognitive evaluation process among other factors, can reduce alcohol consumption directly or facilitate entry into treatment. These brief interventions, often consisting of assessment and advice, are designed to motivate the problem drinker to decrease consumption or become abstinent. They are significantly more effective than no intervention, are frequently as effective if not more effective than extensive intervention, and may increase the effectiveness of subsequent treatment efforts. In reviewing studies of brief interventions, Miller and Sanchez (1994) found that six elements appeared to be common to successful interventions. These included Feedback, Responsibility, Advice, Menu, Empathy, and Self-Efficacy (forming the acronym FRAMES). These components are summarized in table 6.1.

Motivational Interviewing

It has been suggested that brief interventions exert influence on drinking directly or on help seeking by their impact on motivation for change (Miller & Rollnick, 1991). Once this motivational impact has occurred, individuals may change their drinking behavior with or without formal treatment. In their recent book describing motivational interviewing, Miller and Rollnick (1991) indicated that this approach incorporates five principles to guide the therapist: (a) express empathy, (b) develop the client's

TABLE 6.1

Elements in Brief Interventions Shown to be Effective Summarized
by Acronym FRAMES

Feedback of personal risk or impairment
Emphasis on personal **R**esponsibility for change
Clear **A**dvice to change
A **M**enu of alternative change options
Therapeutic **E**mpathy as a counseling style
Enhancement of client **S**elf-efficacy or optimism

Note. From "Brief Interventions for Alcohol Problems: A Review." by T.H. Bien, W.R. Miller, and J.S. Tonigan, 1993, *Addiction, 88,* pp. 326-327.

perceived discrepancy between present behavior and important goals, (c) avoid argumentation, (d) roll with resistance by inviting the client to consider new information and by offering new perspectives, and (e) support self-efficacy by encouraging acceptance of personal responsibility for change and by presenting a range of alternatives for action.

The authors further described motivational strategies that a therapist can use to motivate individuals for change and for treatment. These strategies, arranged alphabetically from A through H for mnemonic purposes, are giving clear *advice* to change, identifying and removing *barriers* to change such as transportation cost or delay in entering treatment, providing *choices* for change strategies and allowing the client to select, decreasing the client's perception of the *desirability* of continued abusive drinking, practicing *empathy* through reflective listening, providing *feedback* regarding the client's current situation and its risks, helping the client to clarify *goals*, and being active in the *helping* relationship (e.g., follow-up phone calls in response to missed appointments, making referral calls).

Motivational interviewing has two phases. Phase I focuses on building motivation for change and incorporates various therapeutic strategies (e.g., open-ended questions, reflective listening) to assist the client in defining the problem and generating sufficient levels of motivation to initiate change. During this stage, resistance to change will likely occur and the therapist must handle it successfully. The authors offer various strategies for the therapist to incorporate in dealing with resistance.

Phase II emphasizes strengthening commitment to change. This process involves helping the client reach a more refined understanding of the problem, entertaining various options for change, selecting and committing to one or more options, and making a transition to the action stage of the process. The authors noted that transition from Phase I to Phase II (in Prochaska et al., 1992, vernacular from contemplation to preparation and action) is a critical window of opportunity for change afforded by discomfort associated with the client's perceived discrepancy between actual (e.g., heavy drinking) and desired (e.g., moderate drinking or abstinence) behavior. Recognizing the window of opportunity and assisting the client to initiate change is the challenge and art of effective therapy. Although the signs of readiness for change vary across individuals and are presently not well researched, table 6.2 lists several cues discussed by the authors. They also discuss potential hazards for the therapist in negotiating Phase II with the client as well as numerous strategies to strengthen the client's commitment to change.

Although these brief motivational interventions may have applications in specialized treatment settings as a cost-effective alternative to more prolonged treatment, perhaps the most promising application of brief motivational counseling is its potential as a low-cost intervention with large populations served in general health, social, employment, and criminal justice settings. This would suggest that nonspecialist health care professionals expecting to have contact with alcohol abusers in their practices (e.g., physicians, nurses, psychologists, social workers, and counselors) could be trained in motivational interviewing strategies to increase their comfort level with this patient or client population and this type of intervention (Miller & Rollnick, 1991). Recent studies suggest that both physicians (Anderson, 1993) and nurses (Rassool, 1993) need education and training in effective early-intervention strategies with alcohol and other substance abusers. The likely result of these applications of motivational interventions is that successful referrals to specialized alcohol treatment would increase and significant reductions in drinking would occur without specialized treatment.

Motivational interventions may accurately be regarded as strategies to assist problem drinkers in successfully negotiating the stages of change necessary to alter their drinking. As

TABLE 6.2

Signs of Readiness for Change

1. **Decreased resistance.** The client stops arguing, interrupting, denying, or objecting.

2. **Decreased questions about the problem.** The client seems to have enough information about his or her problem and stops asking questions. There is a sense of being finished.

3. **Resolve.** The client appears to have reached a resolution and may seem more peaceful, relaxed, calm, unburdened, or settled. Sometimes this happens after the client has passed through a period of anguish or tearfulness.

4. **Self-motivational statements.** The client makes direct self-motivational statements, reflecting recognition of a problem ("I guess this is serious"), concern ("This worries me"), openness to change ("I need to do something"), or optimism ("I'm going to beat this").

5. **Increased questions about change.** The client asks what he or she could do about the problem, how people change if they decide to, or the like.

6. **Envisioning.** The client begins to talk about how life might be after a change, to anticipate difficulties if a change were made, or to discuss the advantages of change.

7. **Experimenting.** If the client has had time between sessions, he or she may have begun experimenting with possible change approaches (e.g., going to an Alcoholics Anonymous meeting, going without drinking for a few days, reading a self-help book).

From *Motivational Interviewing: Preparing People to Change Addictive Behavior* (p. 115) by W. R. Miller and S. Rollnick, 1991, New York: Guilford Press. Copyright 1991 by Guilford Press. Reprinted with permission.

suggested by DiClemente (in Miller & Rollnick, 1991), although these motivational strategies can be effectively used in all stages of change, they may be most appropriate during the early stages of precontemplation, contemplation, and preparation. The following case example of an initial session between an athlete and a psychologist illustrates how motivational intervention strategies might work with an athlete experiencing alcohol-related problems. The case description is for instructional purposes and is modeled after a case example presented in Miller and Rollnick (1991). While reviewing this narrative, pay attention to how the principles of motivational interviewing are reflected in the interviewer's responses to the athlete.

CASE STUDY

Walter

Walter was a 22-year-old college tennis player. He came for consultation about his drinking following two precipitating events. The first was his coach's advice that he seek consultation from a professional for his repeated alcohol-related broken curfews on road trips. The second event was his girlfriend's complaints that his personality changed while he was drinking. He had never sought help for his drinking in the past and appeared to be in the early contemplation stage of change, therefore not at all sure that he needed to make changes to his drinking.

Therapist: Good afternoon. Please have a seat and make yourself comfortable. I understand from our phone conversation that you had some concerns about your drinking. This afternoon I would like to explore with you your situation and some of your concerns. So, please tell me what's been concerning you about your drinking and what led to your coming to see me this afternoon.

Walter: Well, actually I'm not really sure why I'm here. My coach seems to think that I miss too many curfews on road trips and he thinks I drink too much. Also, my girlfriend says I change when I'm drinking, but I don't really understand what she means.

T: So two people who are apparently important to you have been worried about the amount that you are drinking. But I would like to know about what *you* have noticed about your drinking. Have you noticed any changes in your drinking that are causing you concern? Tell me something about how you feel about your drinking.

W: I can't say that I've noticed anything remarkable. I've been drinking since I was in high school. I guess that since being in college I drink more regularly, but I don't really see that it is causing me any problems.

T: You've noticed that you've been drinking more regularly since being in college. What else have you noticed?

W: I guess I probably drink more beers at any one time than I did in high school or during my first couple of years in college. But I don't think that my drinking has caused any serious problems. I mean I don't get drunk very often at all.

(continued)

T: So while you've noticed that you drink more often and usually drink more per occasion, you don't notice that the alcohol affects you any more than it did previously.

W: That's right. The stuff doesn't seem to affect me that much. My friends seem to get a lot drunker than I do.

T: That's interesting. What do you think causes that?

W: I don't know. I guess maybe I have more experience with alcohol. I've been drinking for five or six years and people in my family have always been able to drink a lot without really feeling it.

T: You come from a family with some pretty heavy drinkers.

W: Yeah, my dad, brothers, and I could always put away our share of beer.

T: In what ways has alcohol affected your family members?

W: My dad had a few problems with his liver. He said that his doctor told him that his drinking probably caused some of his liver problems. My dad tells me that my grandfather had a few problems with alcohol before he died.

T: Your father and grandfather seemed to have a few alcohol-related problems. Do you have any other concerns about your own drinking at this time?

W: Occasionally, when I have a few too many the night before, I feel pretty groggy the next morning and I swear that I won't drink that much again. Also, there have been a few times when I couldn't remember exactly how I had gotten home the previous night. That can be a little strange.

T: In what way?

W: Well, it scares me a little when I can't remember what happened the night before. I guess I think I might do something that would hurt me.

T: What are some examples?

W: Oh, maybe get in a fight with someone bigger than me or get in a bad wreck with the car.

T: So, you're concerned that you might hurt yourself or someone else?

W: Yeah, I guess I can handle myself pretty well in most situations but it's a little unnerving when I can't remember.

T: How have you reacted following these situations?

W: I usually tell myself that I won't drink that much again. And I usually go for a long time before something like that happens again.

T: Let me see if I understand what you have told me so far. Sounds like you have noticed several things about your drinking. You seem to have increased your drinking over the last several years, and you know that, like your father and some other family members, you seem to be able to drink more than your friends without feeling the effects. You have indicated that both your coach and girlfriend have expressed concern about your drinking, even though you feel that it's not a cause for concern. You've noticed that occasionally when you drink too much you feel groggy the next morning and have not been able to remember all the events of the preceding evening. While this has been concerning you, for the most part you feel that you can take care of yourself. Of the things that you've mentioned, which seems to concern you the most?

W: I think when I can't remember the night before—that is pretty scary.

T: That doesn't seem very typical to you.

W: No, I don't think it happens to my friends. But I don't think that it is a big problem. I don't think I'm an alcoholic or anything like that.

T: Things don't seem that bad to you then.

W: No, they don't. I feel like I have a pretty good handle on my drinking. I've been times without drinking for several weeks and it doesn't seem to bother me at all. I'm doing pretty good in school and my match records are pretty good this year.

T: Things must seem a little confusing to you. You have your coach and girlfriend expressing concern about your drinking. At the same time, however, you seem to be doing okay and you don't seem to fit the general picture you have in mind for someone who has a drinking problem.

W: That's right. I know I've got some problems like everybody else, but I don't think one of them is alcohol.

T: So you don't think you really need to do anything about your drinking right now. But you have come here this afternoon for this appointment. Why come here now?

(continued)

139

W: It just seemed like the right thing to do. I don't think I have a problem with alcohol, but I didn't want to ignore what my coach and girlfriend were saying.

T: It sounds like they are two important people in your life.

W: They sure are. I hope my relationship with my girlfriend lasts a long time. And my coach has been real good to me in the last four years; I don't want to let him down.

T: Well, they certainly seem to care about you as well. Sometimes it is very difficult for those who really care about us to point out the things that seem to be causing problems.

W: Yeah, I guess you are right.

T: This appointment must have been a difficult one for you to make and keep. I really appreciate your being so open and honest about your situation. I realize that's not always an easy thing to do.

W: I guess it really wasn't all that easy. Several times I almost decided not to come. But do you think I have a problem with my drinking?

T: That's a good question and I'm not really sure we have enough information at this point. What I think is important is that you take some time to look at this issue closely. Based on what you have told me, I can understand why you have some concern. I would like to help you find out more about the risk your drinking potentially poses and what, if anything, you might want to do about it.

W: So what do you think I should do now?

T: What I would recommend is that we meet again to continue our discussion and perhaps explore other ways alcohol may have influenced your life. As I mentioned before, I think it is important that you spend some time really analyzing this situation now. It is certainly better to make some decisions about your drinking while you are young so if you feel that it's necessary you can make some changes to your drinking. The bottom line, however, is that it will be basically left up to you. It is your decision about whether or not your drinking poses any problems for you and also your decision whether or not you want to do anything about those problems at this time.

This case study demonstrates motivational interviewing strategies designed to elicit concerns from the client regarding his or her drinking and to increase discrepancy between his present situation and his perceived objective, which is probably at this point being able to drink without significant related problems. The therapist primarily was attempting to elicit self-motivational statements and by reflective listening reinforcing these statements. Where the interview leaves off is a choice point. The therapist could continue with building motivation by accumulating self-motivational statements that could further enhance discrepancy. A second choice would be to proceed with the Phase II process of strengthening commitment and possibly negotiating a plan for change. This therapist has decided to proceed with motivation building in a subsequent session. This decision depends on the therapeutic situation and the availability of opportunities to continue the counseling process. If appropriately trained as a specialist, the therapist may include more formal and elaborate assessment of this client's alcohol use patterns and consequences of his drinking on his physical, psychological, and social functioning. If the therapist is not trained to provide further specialized treatment, the goal of therapy may be either to encourage the client to change his drinking habits on his own or to establish sufficient self-motivation to pursue specialized treatment in another context. Additional information regarding motivational interviewing and the potential role it may play in the treatment of problem drinkers is available in Miller and Rollnick (1991). This book provides a thorough description of the motivational interview along with background literature substantiating its use. In addition, it provides examples of several clinical applications for motivational interviewing, including motivational interviewing with alcoholic couples, young people, problem drinkers experiencing relapse, and individuals experiencing other addictive behaviors.

CONCLUSION

Problem drinkers resolve their alcohol-related difficulties both with and without treatment. Recent research suggests that problem drinkers move through identifiable stages of change during their recovery. Movement through these stages appears to be predicated on a self-appraisal process, which may occur through or independent from therapist guidance.

In this chapter, we learned that brief interventions that focus on increasing the problem drinker's motivation to change have been effective in reducing alcohol consumption. Specialized and nonspecialized helping professionals have successfully administered these interventions. Certainly, a variety of helping professionals with training in motivational interviewing techniques could have administered the interview conducted in the case study.

Although brief interventions have demonstrated effectiveness in changing problem drinking, many individuals require more extensive, specialized treatment for their alcohol abuse or dependence. For these individuals, motivational interviewing may serve as the impetus for them to enter more extensive treatment. The next chapter describes what the athlete who requires this level of care might encounter.

7 ALCOHOL TREATMENT AND ATHLETES

Alcohol addiction may be the hardest substance abuse problem to treat in athletes "because of team spirit, which has alcohol use embedded in it."

—Joseph A. Pursch, MD

The focus of the previous chapter was primarily on changing drinking behavior in individuals who were in early stages of developing alcohol-related problems. Alcohol treatment specialists could administer the interventions discussed, however, their most valuable application would be in settings (e.g., primary care physicians' offices, university counseling centers, and social service agencies) where helping professionals see clients who would benefit from intervention, although their drinking may not meet diagnostic criteria for abuse or dependence. In contrast, chapter 7 describes treatment that health professionals with specialized addiction treatment training or experience would administer. This chapter educates the reader regarding the characteristics of treatment approaches, the relative effectiveness of various treatment modalities, and methods used to match clients with appropriate treatment interventions. How the sport experience may influence the athlete's treatment seeking and participation, the potential positive transfer of sport-related skills to the tasks confronted in treatment, and issues involved in evaluating and selecting appropriate treatment professionals or organizations for athletes are also discussed.

WHAT IS TREATMENT?

Alcohol treatment has undergone considerable evolution during the past two decades in the United States and is likely to undergo further change as a result of many forces, including treatment research and changes in health care delivery and third party reimbursement. To facilitate an overview of available treatments, it is best to first define treatment. A committee of the Institute of Medicine established a general definition and produced an influential book entitled *Broadening the Base of Treatment for Alcohol Problems* (Institute of Medicine, 1990). This committee's definition is as follows:

> *Treatment refers to the broad range of services, including identification, brief intervention, assessment, diagnosis, counseling, medical services, psychiatric services, psychological services, social services, and follow-up, for persons with alcohol problems. The goal of treatment is to reduce or eliminate the use of alcohol as a contributing factor to phys-*

ical, psychological, and social dysfunction and to arrest, retard, or reverse the progress of any associated problems. (Institute of Medicine, 1990, p. 46)

This definition includes a variety of treatment activities that form a continuum of services to meet the needs of individuals experiencing problems with alcohol, whether they be minimal, moderate, or severe.

Three major orientations have been recognized as foundations for modalities used in the treatment of alcohol problems: physiological, psychological, and sociocultural (Armor, Polich, & Stambul, 1978; Saxe, Dougherty, Esty, & Fine, 1983). These orientations reflect ideological positions of various treatment professionals about the etiology and appropriate treatment of alcohol problems. Although each orientation has historical value, it is their integration that has yielded the approach frequently used in contemporary treatment programs. This orientation is typically labeled the biopsychosocial approach because it takes into account that all three factors may be involved to varying degrees in the alcohol problems of an individual. In this approach, the etiology, maintenance, and consequences of alcohol problems are seen as the product of an interaction between physiological (or biological), psychological, and sociocultural factors. For example, physiological factors might include genetic predispositions that increase an individual's risk for alcohol problems; psychological factors may include personality characteristics and expectations regarding the effects of alcohol; and sociocultural factors may include social, family, and work-environment variables that influence drinking behavior.

The most influential model for alcohol treatment in the United States is what has become known as the Minnesota model, which is a treatment approach that combines professional input with the guidelines of Alcoholics Anonymous (AA) (Spicer, 1993). Although the Minnesota model has yet to receive strong empirical support because of the lack of available research on its effectiveness, it has served as the basis for most treatment programs in both the public and private sectors. The treatment program advocated by the Minnesota model often includes detoxification, education based on the disease concept of alcoholism, confrontation, AA meeting attendance, and use of AA materials to devise a recovery plan (*step work*), among other interventions

(Institute of Medicine, 1990). The Minnesota model will be discussed later in this chapter with stages of care.

MODALITIES OF CARE

As noted earlier, many alcoholics recover without formal treatment or intervention. Although we don't fully understand this process of self-recovery, it appears that individuals who can stop drinking without treatment undergo a process of self-appraisal that contributes to their decision to discontinue drinking (see section in chapter 6 on facilitating change in problem drinkers). Self-help groups may be effective for some individuals; however, a recent review of these approaches suggested that habit disturbances such as smoking, drinking, and overeating may be more difficult to change through self-help methods than other problems, such as fears, depression, and sleep disturbance (Gould & Clum, 1993).

Professional help for alcohol-related problems takes various forms and intensities. Most communities have professionals available who are capable of helping individuals with drinking problems. These professionals come from a variety of backgrounds, including medicine, psychology, social work, nursing, counseling, and vocational rehabilitation. Professionals will vary in their approach to treating an individual with alcohol problems. Some professionals will teach self-control skills to assist the individual in altering their drinking patterns. Others may approach treatment strictly with a goal of abstinence. In addition to services rendered, professionals also may refer clients to some type of self-help group (e.g., Alcoholics Anonymous, Adult Children of Alcoholics, Rational Recovery).

We can divide professional assistance into two types: (a) pharmacological treatment, which includes drugs used to manage withdrawal from alcohol and in long-term rehabilitation, and (b) psychological treatment, which includes approaches with behavioral or psychodynamic orientations. Comprehensive treatment programs will employ both of these types of care as needed.

Pharmacological Treatment

Withdrawal from alcohol usually manifests as a self-limited cluster of symptoms that occurs following a period of heavy drinking.

A person in mild withdrawal may experience anxiety, hand tremors, irritability, sweating, increased heart rate, nausea, vomiting, diarrhea, and sleep disturbance. Onset of these symptoms may be within hours of the last drink. The symptoms usually peak at one or two days following drinking cessation and gradually disappear after three to seven days. A small percentage of persons will experience more severe withdrawal symptoms, which may include seizures or delirium tremens (DTs), a syndrome characterized by profound confusion and disorientation, hyperactivity, and hallucinations.

Withdrawal symptoms are typically managed with benzodiazepines (e.g., Librium, Ativan), which are antianxiety drugs. These drugs reduce the severity of symptoms during withdrawal and are typically terminated after withdrawal symptoms subside. This treatment process is often referred to as medical detoxification and usually takes place in a hospital setting, although recent evidence suggests that medical detoxification can be safely carried out in an ambulatory setting for patients with mild-to-moderate withdrawal symptoms (Hayashida et al., 1989). Nonmedical (social) detoxification also has been carried out successfully. Patients are not given medication but are counseled on what to expect during withdrawal and given emotional and social support, good food, and pleasant surroundings to assist them (see review by Institute of Medicine, 1990).

During rehabilitation, an alcohol-sensitizing drug is often used that results in unpleasant symptoms (e.g., flushing, nausea) when an individual consumes alcohol. The most common medication used for this purpose in the United States is disulfiram (Antabuse). In a recent review of supervised (dose taken by patient while observed by supervisor aware of potential evasion techniques) disulfiram treatment, Brewer (1993) indicated that it is "one of the few demonstrably effective interventions in alcoholism [treatment], both alone and as an adjunct to psychosocial methods" (p. 383). He noted further that despite its apparent effectiveness (when administered under appropriate supervision), especially for those patients not responding to other treatment modalities or for those who would be devastated by an early relapse, supervised disulfiram is underused.

Psychotropic medications also are used during rehabilitation to treat psychopathology associated with drinking. These medications have included antidepressant and antianxiety drugs.

There is ongoing controversy regarding use of the latter drugs because many antianxiety medications also have dependence-producing properties (e.g., Valium). Criteria to evaluate the appropriateness of antianxiety drugs to use during rehabilitation include (a) low potential for abuse, (b) effects on retention of individuals in treatment, and (c) lack of potentiation of alcohol's effects (Institute of Medicine, 1990).

Psychological Treatment

Psychological treatment modalities also take various forms but generally can be categorized as either behavioral or psychodynamic approaches. Behavioral treatments either directly alter drinking behavior or focus on changing related behaviors that may contribute to or result from the drinking. Behavioral approaches include aversion therapies, self-control training, marital and family therapies, stress management and social skills training, contingency management, and relapse prevention strategies. These approaches are often used in various combinations. For the interested reader, a recent book entitled *Handbook of Alcohol Treatment Approaches: Effective Alternatives* (Hester & Miller, 1989) reviews these behavioral treatment approaches.

Psychodynamic modalities for treatment of alcohol problems come in a variety of theoretical orientations and are usually designed to help the individual alter unhelpful thoughts, feelings, and behaviors. If an alcohol problem has existed for sufficient time, usually there are related problems that need treatment attention. These may include marital and family, interpersonal, legal, and employment problems. Both psychodynamic and behavioral modalities may take the form of individual, marital and family, or group therapy. Both modalities also are frequently combined to respond to variable treatment needs among individuals. A brief review of psychodynamic modalities may be found in the Institute of Medicine's 1990 book entitled *Broadening the Base of Treatment for Alcohol Problems* (p. 81).

TREATMENT SETTINGS AND INTENSITIES

Just as a variety of treatment modalities and professionals treat individuals with alcohol problems, the activities involved in treatment may occur in a variety of settings. In general, treatment is provided in one of four settings: inpatient, residential, intermediate, and outpatient (Institute of Medicine, 1990).

- Inpatient settings typically provide 24-hour supervision in a hospital-type setting with services including medical, nursing, counseling, and other support. Treatment is often provided in inpatient settings for detoxification and initial stages of rehabilitation.
- Residential treatment settings provide similar services to inpatient programs, typically with less intensity of medical services.
- Intermediate care facilities provide similar services to inpatient and residential settings; however, services are rendered on a less than 24-hour basis. Intermediate care (also called day treatment) provides services in a setting that is less intensive than inpatient or residential care, yet more intensive and supportive than a typical outpatient setting.
- Outpatient service delivery may include a full spectrum of professional services but treatment is typically less frequent and intensive than in other settings. Outpatient services are often delivered to clients who have completed more intensive treatment in another setting. When services are delivered in this manner it is often referred to as aftercare.

Recent evidence has suggested that less intensive treatment may be as beneficial as more intensive and prolonged treatment (Miller & Hester, 1986a, 1986b). The choice of treatment setting depends on a variety of factors, including the severity of the alcohol abuse and its concomitant problems, the ability of the individual to access a particular type of treatment setting, the existence of environmental support for treatment goals, and the client's motivation to change and to seek help in doing so.

STAGES OF CARE

Successful treatment of individuals with alcohol problems requires meeting both acute and long-term treatment needs. Although several treatment models and stages have been proposed, most are similar and include three stages or phases of treatment that subsume important treatment activities. These stages are acute intervention, rehabilitation, and maintenance (Institute of Medicine, 1990).

Acute Intervention

The acute intervention stage includes treatments designed to resolve immediate medical and psychosocial problems caused by alcohol abuse. These services might include medically supervised detoxification and crisis intervention counseling, which people with severe alcohol problems are likely to need. Also included in this stage are screening activities to identify individuals with alcohol problems and to facilitate a referral to treatment. Screening is usually designed to identify persons with mild or moderate alcohol problems, but it also may detect individuals with severe alcohol problems who may not have been previously identified.

Rehabilitation

The rehabilitation stage assists the client in reducing or eliminating alcohol consumption and attaining improved physical, psychological, and social status. This treatment stage includes comprehensive assessment of the client's current functioning and the development of a treatment plan to address issues that have contributed to or resulted from the drinking problem. Following evaluation, primary care occurs in which therapeutic activities assist the client in changing drinking patterns and beginning to resolve related problems. A period of extended care (stabilization) occurs after primary care, including continued treatment participation and various supportive activities (e.g., participation in self-help groups) to consolidate gains made during primary care. The length of both primary and extended care for an individual depends on the degree of severity of their problems. All or part of the rehabilitation stage may occur in any of the treatment settings: inpatient, residential, intermediate, or outpatient.

Maintenance

The maintenance stage includes activities to maintain treatment gains made during primary and extended care. These activities are known as aftercare and relapse prevention, and many treatment professionals regard them as pivotal to the individual's ability to sustain long-term sobriety. This treatment stage may also include provision of treatment services in a domiciliary setting for those individuals unable to return to independent living in the community.

These stages of care represent a continuum of care necessary to provide sufficient services to meet the needs of individuals with alcohol problems of varying degrees of severity. As an individual progresses through these stages of care, it is important to evaluate progress at entry and exit from each stage. Depending on the individual's progress and on relapse to alcohol use, reentry into previous treatment stages may be necessary, along with a change in the setting or modality of treatment.

WHAT TREATMENT WORKS?

Gaining insight into treatments that work most effectively for alcohol abusers is a frequently misguided endeavor or ignored completely. Research has suggested that many professionals and the general public in the United States labor under common beliefs about the nature of and recovery from alcohol problems that current empirical evidence does not substantiate (Miller, 1990). These common but unsupported beliefs about treatment are (a) no one is able to recover from alcohol problems without treatment, (b) no treatment for alcoholism works, (c) all treatments are equally efficacious, (d) there is one treatment approach or method that is superior to all others, and (e) treatment occurring in hospital settings is the most effective. Recent reviews of the literature (Miller & Hester, 1986a, 1986b, 1986c) have indicated that many treatment programs in the United States have been based on these unsupported ideas regarding alcohol problems and the recovery process. Miller (1990) reached six conclusions that this treatment literature supports. These conclusions are as follows:

1. There is reason for optimism regarding some alcohol treatment approaches as evidenced by positive clinical trials, which have shown significant treatment effects.

2. There is no evidence for one superior approach to treatment, but rather a number of promising alternatives that have demonstrated effectiveness.

3. Not all treatment approaches have equal effectiveness. Controlled clinical trials have supported a finite number of

treatment strategies falling into two categories: alcohol-suppressing and broad-spectrum strategies. The first category consists of strategies that directly suppress alcohol consumption and includes aversion therapies, behavioral self-control training, and monitored disulfiram. The second category, often referred to as broad spectrum, includes strategies that target life issues or problems besides drinking that may functionally relate to alcohol use. The aim of these interventions is to prevent further drinking by assisting the individual to cope with problems that may trigger a relapse to drinking. Strategies in this category that have received consistent experimental support are social skills training, behavioral marital therapy, stress management, and the community reinforcement approach (see table 7.1 for explanations of both categories of treatment approaches). Other treatment approaches have shown promise but have not received as much support, perhaps because they are new or present difficulties in accurately evaluating their effects. These include relapse prevention, self-help groups, psychotropic medications, and brief interventions. As discussed in chapter 6, brief interventions have recently received experimental support in numerous controlled studies, suggesting that well-planned brief interventions are effective in altering harmful drinking patterns (Bien, Miller, & Tonigan, 1993). Unfortunately, as Miller (1990) noted, current U.S. treatment programs infrequently use treatment strategies that the scientific literature supports. He argued that incorporating treatment approaches that have demonstrated effectiveness can improve efficacy of alcoholism treatment.

4. Problem drinkers are a heterogeneous population and will respond differently to various treatment approaches. Therefore, treatment programs should be tailored to fit the characteristics of the individuals being treated. Also, treatment should address the broad spectrum of problems often associated with alcohol abuse, in addition to the drinking behavior.

5. Treatment length, intensity, and setting do not appear to be strong determining factors of effectiveness. The strongest determining factor appears to be *what* is done with clients rather than where it is done, with what frequency

TABLE 7.1

Treatment Approaches Supported by Controlled Clinical Trials

Aversion therapies—designed to reduce desire for alcohol and to develop a distaste of drinking through conditioned aversion.

Behavioral self-control training—involves teaching self-control strategies to assist clients in modifying their drinking.

Disulfiram—medication taken daily causing person to have unpleasant reaction if alcohol is consumed. Program to ensure compliance is needed for effectiveness.

Social skills training—involves training in communication skills, assertiveness, and dealing with peer pressure.

Behavioral marital therapy—focuses on improving couples' communication strategies and increasing the quality of shared experiences.

Stress management—involves teaching skills to reduce tension and anxiety, including systematic desensitization, aerobic exercise, and biofeedback.

Community reinforcement approach—combines various broad-spectrum strategies including training in job finding and problem solving, behavioral marital therapy, monitored disulfiram.

From "Alcohol Treatment Alternatives: What Works?" by W.R. Miller. In *Treatment Choices for Alcoholism and Substance Abuse* (pp. 256-258) by H.B. Milkman and L.I. Sederer (Eds.), 1990, New York: Lexington Books.

it occurs, or how long it lasts. The literature supports the idea that brief interventions on an outpatient basis can alter harmful drinking patterns and often can be at least as effective as more extensive and costly treatment options.

6. Therapist style and characteristics directly relate to treatment effectiveness. Although a confrontational therapist style has been typical in alcoholism treatment historically in the United States, it has been shown recently that this style may be counterproductive, leading to increases in client resistance and to poorer long term treatment outcomes than an empathic, supportive (client-centered) style (Miller, Benefield, & Tonigan, 1993).

MATCHING CLIENT NEEDS WITH TREATMENT PROGRAMS

Recent research supports the idea that individuals with alcohol-related problems can be matched to various interventions to increase treatment effectiveness (which supports Miller's conclusion #4 *above*). For instance, Babor et al. (1992) found that alcoholics may be divided effectively into subtypes to match clients to appropriate treatments, which yield more favorable treatment outcomes than clients that are mismatched (Litt, Babor, DelBoca, Kadden, & Cooney, 1992). These recent studies have indicated that client-treatment matching based on client characteristics has validity. However, presently there are no clear guidelines, or perhaps rudimentary ones at best, upon which to base this matching process. In addition, effective matching requires the availability of a variety of treatment options, which in most areas is not the case.

Because matching clients to treatments has inherent benefits as noted by Miller (1989b), in the absence of substantiated guidelines for matching, how might this process be accomplished? One option, which has intuitive as well as empirical support, is for therapists to assist clients through negotiation to self-select or match themselves into an appropriate treatment. As described by Miller, this process would include the therapist presenting a *menu* of known treatment alternatives to the client and information regarding the probable outcomes of the treatment alternatives, given the client's individual characteristics. The outcome of the negotiation process ideally would be the client making an informed and appropriate decision about treatment.

Tentative guidelines for this negotiation and decision-making process are diagrammed in figure 7.1. The process involves four levels of matching or decision making, preceded by a comprehensive assessment of the client's needs and followed by an assessment of treatment outcome.

- Level 1 is a negotiation of treatment goals, which will typically entail goals involving alcohol use, other drug use, and other life problems, such as marital, legal, or mood problems.

- Level 2 is agreeing on the intensity of intervention, varying from no intervention needed to residential or inpatient treatment. Guiding this second level of negotiation is the

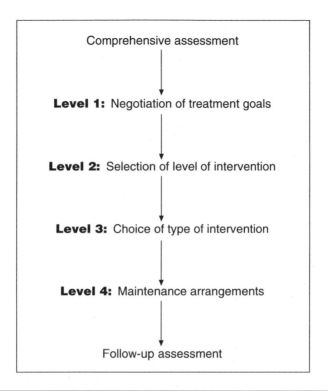

Comprehensive assessment

Level 1: Negotiation of treatment goals

Level 2: Selection of level of intervention

Level 3: Choice of type of intervention

Level 4: Maintenance arrangements

Follow-up assessment

Figure 7.1 The process of matching.

From "Matching Individuals with Interventions" by W.R. Miller. In *Handbook of Alcoholism Treatment Approaches: Effective Alternatives* (p.264), by R. K. Hester and W. R. Miller (Eds.), 1989, New York: Pergamon Press. Copyright 1989 W.R. Miller. Adapted with permission.

principle that the least intensive treatment meeting the client's needs and goals should be tried first, with more supervised care to follow if treatment at the lesser intensity level is unsuccessful.

- Level 3 is a selection of type of intervention. Interventions typically either focus on altering drinking patterns or remedying problems contributing to or resulting from drinking (broad-spectrum intervention). Because there is limited current knowledge of how to match individuals' characteristics with specific treatment types, other indices of an appropriate match should be used. These might include clients' compliance and satisfaction with treatment and their early treatment response.

- Level 4 is arranging continued contact following formal treatment termination. Options vary in intensity and content and, as with the preceding three levels, the therapist should present them and make decisions relying on client input, experience, and other available information. The appropriateness and effectiveness of the maintenance arrangement can be judged as in Level 3 by clients' compliance and satisfaction and their early responses to it regarding maintaining gains made in treatment.

A follow-up assessment is completed to determine the overall effectiveness of the interventions selected. This assessment may be done through mail, telephone, or face-to-face contact with clients and their family members or other significant people in their lives (e.g., friends, employers, probation officers). The assessment may also be used to gain valuable information from the client or others on what intervention components were most helpful. Also, the follow-up contact may have direct impact on the client by providing access to a treatment professional who offers services or referral if the client is experiencing difficulties. The assessment may be done by the treatment provider or by some independent entity, the latter being preferable if objectivity of results is valued. The importance of this follow-up cannot be overestimated, for it is only through this assessment that improvements in treatment may be made. Interested readers are referred to Miller (1989a) for additional information on follow-up assessment.

TREATMENT IMPLICATIONS FOR ATHLETES

Athletes with alcohol problems will come to treatment with many therapeutic issues similar to those of the general population. After all, athletes are a subset of the general population that frequently mirrors many of the health-related behaviors of the larger group. This is particularly the case with alcohol use. Therefore, athletes should receive the same treatment alternatives as the general population with the expectation that treatment outcomes would be essentially the same. However, the sport experience also may alter treatment and either facilitate or detract from the process. The following sections discuss ways in which sport may affect treatment.

Sport Experience and Alcohol Treatment

It is important to address how the sport experience influences the athlete's seeking and participating in treatment. Because treatment typically progresses through three stages, it should be helpful to examine how sport participation may influence progression through these stages of treatment. As described previously, during the acute intervention stage, individuals receive treatment services designed to identify and establish the existence of an alcohol problem and to resolve acute, alcohol-related medical or psychosocial problems. This treatment may include detoxification and crisis intervention counseling. Because athletes usually are in superior physical condition relative to the general population, they may be able to withstand longer and heavier drinking bouts before requiring medical attention, therefore delaying the acute intervention stage of treatment. Conversely, because their athletic performance depends on maintaining conditioning, the physical effects of alcohol may be more apparent and detectable for the athlete, which may precipitate the acute intervention stage of treatment more rapidly than for the average person. Health professionals in a position to diagnose an athlete with an alcohol problem must be aware that sport participation may either delay or facilitate entry into the acute intervention stage of treatment.

During the rehabilitation stage, an important treatment activity is a comprehensive assessment of the physical, psychological, and social factors that have both determined and resulted from the athlete's alcohol abuse. It is also a stage in which treatment should focus on helping the athlete reduce or discontinue alcohol use and attain more adaptive levels of functioning. Depending on whether the athlete is in a competitive season, this stage of treatment may pose significant disruption to the athlete's activities. Even if not in a competitive season, participation in rehabilitation requires the athlete's commitment of both time and energy, which must come from other parts of the athlete's life. Although the outcome of treatment in terms of mental and physical well-being may compensate for the time and effort expended, the athlete must still make the decision initially that the alcohol problem warrants treatment and that the effort is worth the projected outcome. Depending on the athlete's situation regarding competition and practice demands, the therapist may need to devote extra attention to motivation for treatment.

Maintenance Stage of Treatment and Long-Term Outcome

In the maintenance stage of treatment the therapeutic goals are maintaining treatment gains realized during rehabilitation and preventing a return to drinking and related behavior patterns. Many professionals believe that this stage of treatment is the most important in determining the long-term outcome of the treatment process. It is during this stage that the individual must confront the environmental factors that played significant contributing roles in the drinking problem. These factors will differ with the individual but often include family, employment, and interpersonal issues.

The athlete may face numerous issues in the maintenance stage that represent significant challenges. For instance, he or she must reestablish training and competitive routines, which might include significant physical and mental expenditures, to reclaim former competitive levels. Of course, this demand will vary depending on how much disruption to training the rehabilitation phase causes. For less severe alcohol problems, the athlete may spend limited or no time away from training or competition. For severe alcohol problems, the time spent away from competition may be significant. During the maintenance stage, the athlete faces potentially altered relationships with coaches, teammates, family members, and so forth, who may be uncertain about how to respond to the individual because his or her behavior will likely be substantially different from before treatment. The magnitude of this adjustment also will depend on the severity of the alcohol problem and the level of intervention required in the rehabilitation phase.

It is likely that athletes in the maintenance stage will have to contend with slips in which they might deviate from their alcohol-related treatment goal of abstinence or nonproblem drinking. These slips occur in most people seeking to change an addictive behavior and should not be regarded as a failure but as an expected part of the change process. The athlete can most constructively view it as an opportunity to learn from the slip and return to the treatment goal that was established, whether it be abstinence or a reduction in drinking.

Finally, the maintenance stage of treatment may require athletes to maintain contact with professionals or self-help groups over an extended time, the length of which depends on their progress in reaching treatment goals. Athletes who must travel during their competitive seasons may have difficulty accessing professional help; however, self-help groups are typically available throughout the United States and in many foreign countries.

Positive Transfer From Sport to Treatment

By virtue of their sport experience, athletes often bring to the treatment process particular skills that contribute positively to changing their drinking-related behaviors. Developed over many years in sport, athletes could use these skills during their recovery from problem drinking and beyond. Examples of these skills are discussed below.

1. Athletes may have well-developed skills to set and work toward goals. During their sport careers, most athletes have had to develop personal mechanisms to establish realistic goals for themselves and methods to attain them. This ability may serve a useful purpose, particularly when negotiating treatment goals and interventions.

2. Athletes may have the ability to assess athletic strengths and weaknesses and develop plans to capitalize on strengths and improve weaknesses. Although this ability may not transfer directly to endeavors outside of sport, with therapeutic assistance, the athlete may learn how to adapt this athletic ability to assist in the treatment process.

3. Athletes may be able to self-reward incremental progress toward goals and thereby enhance confidence. Resolving an alcohol problem is typically not an all-or-nothing event. The change process is characterized by successes and relapses, which must be learned from and overcome. To the extent athletes can self-reward progress in making adaptive changes to drinking, they will enhance their recovery.

4. Athletes may have the ability to manage time so they can accomplish both athletic and other life goals. Most athletic careers are characterized by multiple demands placed on time and energy. To succeed, athletes must find ways to manage their time effectively to meet both athletic and other life demands. For many individuals recovering from an alcohol problem, effective time management often becomes an issue in treatment. When drinking is

removed or diminished as an alternative in the problem drinker's repertoire of activities, an important challenge for the individual becomes using the time previously spent drinking for other activities. This issue often takes the form of striking a reasonable balance between work and leisure time.

5. Athletes may be able to focus attention on tasks at hand and follow through until they complete the tasks. For most athletes, success has depended on their ability to focus on perfecting skills that have required many hours of repetitive practice. Progress may be inconsistent, demanding patience and tenacity on the part of the athlete. This experience is not unlike the demands faced by individuals changing drinking behaviors. Progress during recovery will depend on the individual developing a sense of purpose, learning strategies to cope effectively without alcohol, and implementing these strategies to shape a different lifestyle not dependent on alcohol.

6. Athletes may have the ability to accept direction and guidance (coaching) to improve athletic performance. Throughout their careers athletes have received coaching to assist them in skill development and in motivation to improve. While in treatment, the athlete will likely be involved in individual or group therapy, assisting them in skill development to modify their drinking and to sustain motivation to maintain these changes. This work with a therapist in many ways is analogous to the athlete's previous relationships with coaches. If the athlete can realize and capitalize on the similarities in the relationships, the treatment process may be enhanced.

7. Athletes may be able to accept and to live with competitive pressures and the often high expectations of others. The careers of athletes take place in competitive and highly visible circumstances with expectations of others frequently beyond reasonable levels. To thrive under these conditions, athletes must not only be able to accept their existence but also be prepared to establish self-esteem and confidence apart from their athletic performance. In treatment for alcohol problems, the individual has a similar task. They seek to change a behavior (problem drinking) that is difficult to change, where slips or mistakes are highly visible, and where the expectations of others

are frequently beyond reasonable levels (e.g., assuming that stopping or changing drinking is easy and should only require will power). To successfully change a drinking problem, the athlete might draw valuable lessons from the athletic experience, particularly as it relates to establishing internally based self-esteem and dealing effectively with frequently unreasonable expectations of others.

To the extent that the athlete comes to treatment with these attributes, the treatment process may be facilitated. On the other hand, many athletes either have not developed these skills or have lost the ability to selectively apply them in the context of their alcohol problem. In this instance, the treatment process can help to either develop or restore these skills so the individual can apply them not only in athletics but also in other life pursuits.

SELECTING TREATMENT RESOURCES FOR ATHLETES

For those individuals in a position to identify and refer athletes to alcohol treatment (e.g., helping professionals, coaches, sport administrators), it is important to understand what to look for in a potential treatment resource. Because a variety of professionals and organizations are involved in alcohol treatment, an effective referral will take some knowledge of many potential treatment resources. The following paragraphs address specific issues that are important in determining how best to evaluate and select a treatment professional or organization to manage athletes with alcohol problems.

1. A professional should perform a comprehensive evaluation to determine the nature and severity of the athlete's alcohol problem. This evaluation should include not only alcohol-related issues but also other factors that may have contributed to or resulted from alcohol use. A professional conducting this evaluation may come from a variety of backgrounds (psychology, psychiatry, social work, medicine, counseling), and in many cases a combination of professionals may complete the evaluation. A related issue is whether the evaluators are independent from the potential treatment providers. Ideally, those who eval-

uate should be free to make referral decisions without attachment to any particular treatment organization or philosophy. What is most important is that the professionals be knowledgeable of alcohol problems and the treatment options available.

2. A treatment resource should have multiple, documented treatment options available that accommodate various levels of alcohol problem severity and client characteristics. Research reviewed previously indicates that individuals with alcohol problems represent a heterogeneous population and respond differently to various treatment approaches. Therefore, a singular treatment approach for all individuals is inappropriate. It is important to determine not only if various treatment approaches are available but also whether there are efforts made to match patients with these treatment modalities accordingly. Although many programs have similar components of treatment (e.g., group therapy, educational seminars), clients should receive treatment that addresses their issues, not a standard protocol. Whether individualized treatment is actually delivered is best judged by discussing the treatment experience with the athlete and with the professional responsible for developing the comprehensive treatment plan.

3. A follow-up assessment of outcome should be completed on each client. As described by Miller (1989a), a follow-up assessment is "a systematic, structured, individual contact at one or more designated intervals following treatment" (p. 81). Ideally, this assessment should determine the effectiveness of treatment in altering the client's drinking behavior and in resolving related problems. In addition, to the extent that independent and external agents conduct this assessment, the validity of the results will increase. Results from follow-up evaluation will not only give insight into the impact of treatment for the individual but also will indicate the effectiveness of the program so future referrals can be made appropriately.

Other issues that may be answered readily regarding a treatment resource are whether the program is accredited by the Joint Commission of Accreditation of Hospital Organizations (JCAHO), whether there is a balance of professional and recovering staff members, and whether athletes that have been treated by a particular organization or professional have responded well and are doing well after treatment. Selecting appropriate treatment resources for athletes often requires some patience and persistence. Alcohol treatment has become a large business, with programs having various degrees of quality and professionalism. Time spent becoming familiar with treatment options before needing them may prevent unnecessary delays when treatment is needed and will increase the likelihood that appropriate care is delivered in the most effective and cost-efficient manner.

CONCLUSION

As demonstrated in this chapter, there are a broad range of services that fit under the rubric of alcohol treatment. For the helping professional attempting to refer an athlete for specialized care for an alcohol-related problem, the options for care may be confusing. Therefore, perhaps the most important task for the referring professional is to develop a relationship with a professional resource able to perform a thorough evaluation to determine the nature and severity of the athlete's alcohol problem and through negotiation with the athlete decide on the most appropriate treatment (varying in modality, setting, and intensity). This resource should be knowledgeable of the breadth of treatment available and should be able to refer athletes to appropriate treatment based on their current needs. Also, it is important that this professional resource be readily available because athletes experiencing alcohol problems frequently present to a health professional with some type of emergent (e.g., family crisis, legal problems, withdrawal symptoms) situation, which often represents an advantageous time for professional evaluation and treatment. Remember that much depends on this professional's judgment, most importantly, the welfare of the athlete. Therefore, spend time evaluating the professional's skills and reliability.

8 CONCLUSIONS AND FUTURE CONSIDERATIONS

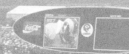

The real voyage of discovery consists not in seeking new landscapes but in having new eyes.

—Marcel Proust

This chapter will provide a brief summary and concluding remarks along with considerations of what role sport professionals may play in minimizing the potential negative consequences of alcohol use in sport and society.

ALCOHOL AND ADDICTION

Alcohol is the most used psychoactive drug in many cultures. Approximately two-thirds of the population in the United States are alcohol consumers with roughly 9 percent of the adult population experiencing alcohol abuse or dependence. Although there have been recent declines in alcohol consumption in the United States, alcohol is still the major drug of abuse. American men are more likely to drink and to drink heavily than American women. Problems related to alcohol use occur with various levels of severity and occur in a wide spectrum of drinkers; however, a composite description of a heavy drinker is male, aged 18–29, and single.

Alcohol abuse is associated with significant medical and psychiatric morbidity and mortality. Alcohol is the third leading, nongenetic contributor to death behind tobacco use and diet and activity patterns.

Risk factors for alcohol dependence have been categorized along biological, psychological, and social lines. A family history of alcohol dependence has been shown to be the most powerful predictor of alcohol dependence in an individual. However, the composite picture of the at-risk individual also includes a predisposing psychiatric disorder such as a conduct disorder, hyperactivity, or generalized anxiety, and a high-risk social environment that provides easy access to alcohol or perhaps encourages membership in a peer group that values alcohol consumption. Despite the presence of numerous biopsychosocial risk factors for alcohol dependence, our ability to predict which individuals will develop alcohol problems is limited.

Though there are multiple costs to society related to alcohol use, its use is part of our cultural custom and therefore is likely to continue. The majority of people consume alcohol without negative consequences; however, many Americans experience abuse- or dependence-related problems that adversely affect themselves, their families, and society. The task of minimizing these adverse effects of alcohol abuse is monumental, ongoing, and will fall partly to professionals and participants involved in sport.

ALCOHOL USE IN SPORT

The strong association between alcohol, particularly beer, and sport has been demonstrated. Underlying this relationship is an apparent high correlation between the demographics of beer drinkers and of sports fans, which has prompted beer breweries to concentrate their marketing efforts in sport. This correlation has promoted a symbiotic relationship between breweries and sport organizations whereby the ever-increasing finances associated with sports (e.g., professional players' salaries, event costs, etc.) strengthen the relationship between the alcohol and sport industries because advertising and sponsorship dollars provided by breweries are more highly valued by sport organizations.

Data from various studies of athlete alcohol use at the secondary-school, collegiate/amateur, and professional levels suggest that athletes' alcohol use is similar to their age and sex mates in the general population. There also are some data and an abundance of anecdotal evidence that athletes may consume alcohol more frequently and to excess than the general population.

Alcohol use by sport professionals is considered in this chapter due to the potential impact of drinking among these professionals on their skill and willingness to identify problem drinking in athletes. Because literature on alcohol use by coaches and sport administrators is scarce, general population data on alcohol use are the best estimates for these sport professionals. Available data on alcohol use by health professionals (e.g., physicians and nurses) indicates that their drinking approximates the general population with some exceptions. For instance, some studies have found that alcohol consumption increases with age among male physicians, which is unlike the general population. Given the critical nature of their duties, this level of alcohol use among physicians may be of concern.

Alcohol use by spectators at sporting events is evidently commonplace. Recent tragedies associated with fan alcohol use involving violence among fans and directed toward players and property have been a solemn documentation of the problems created by heavy drinking at athletic events. Recently, sport administrators are taking precautions to reduce the likelihood of these alcohol-related problems.

Information contained in chapter 2 suggests that the alcohol-sport connection was created and will likely be maintained by a variety of factors. Whether this relationship is negative or positive is not really the issue. What is more important is how the relationship can be properly managed to minimize the potential negative consequences of alcohol abuse.

ALCOHOL, HUMAN FUNCTIONING, AND SPORT PERFORMANCE

Alcohol is a drug that is absorbed unaltered, rapidly, and directly into the body and distributed throughout body fluids, tissues, and organs. It has numerous acute pharmacological effects many of which may influence sport performance. These pharmacological effects are reviewed in chapter 3 along with the effects of alcohol on organ systems and on behavior. Laboratory- and field-based studies on the alcohol–human performance relationship indicate that performance is impaired in a dose-dependent fashion (i.e., as BAC increases, performance decreases). As documented by the ACSM position stand, studies of the effects of alcohol on sport-related performance essentially indicate that alcohol has negative effects on psychomotor performance, little or no beneficial effects (and sometimes negative effects) on metabolic and physiological functions important to physical performance, and no effects or negative effects on muscular work capacity. Light drinking (i.e., one drink) the night before physical performance does not appear to influence physical performance the following morning; however, heavier drinking may decrease performance, particularly in events requiring aerobic conditioning. Furthermore, there are significant interindividual differences in response to alcohol, making it difficult to predict how alcohol will affect an individual's performance.

Given the numerous physical and behavioral effects of alcohol that potentially may influence sport performance, it is important that athletes be educated with regard to the effects of alcohol on physical performance as well as educated regarding individual risk factors for alcohol abuse. While many educational articles regarding alcohol have been published in sport-related trade publications, the need for this educational effort is currently and will likely always be high.

ALCOHOL ABUSE AND DEPENDENCE AMONG ATHLETES AND SPORT PROFESSIONALS

Individuals involved in sport share similar risk factors for alcohol abuse and dependence as the general population as well as risk factors that may be inherent in their sport-related activities. Most research has suggested that the incidence of alcohol abuse and dependence among athletes and sport professionals approximates their peers in the general population. While this may be considered good news by some, this level of problem drinking may be unfortunate news not only for the athletes and sport professionals and their families who experience these problems, but also for the general population whose alcohol-related attitudes and behaviors may be adversely influenced by those of athletes and sport professionals.

Numerous case studies providing descriptive examples of alcohol-abusing and dependent athletes and sport professionals are presented in chapter 4. Key issues exemplified by the case studies and important to helping professionals dealing with problem-drinking athletes include an awareness of the continuum of severity that exists in alcohol-related problems, the ambivalence about changing drinking practices that is often a characteristic of problem drinkers, and the importance of confidentiality to effective helping relationships with athletes seeking assistance for drinking problems. Other important issues reviewed include identifying problems that frequently coexist with alcohol abuse and dependence, exploring multiple sources of diagnostic information, being knowledgeable of potential constraints on the validity of client self-report, understanding the importance of monitoring alcohol and drug use with breathalyzers and urine drug screens, and being aware of minimum age drinking laws.

SPORT-RELATED ALCOHOL ABUSE AND DEPENDENCE PREVENTION

The tremendous human and financial costs associated with alcohol abuse and dependence more than justify the funds expended on alcohol abuse prevention programs. Prevention strategies have been grouped as targeting individual and environmental factors that influence alcohol use and contribute to increased risk for alcohol problems. Since both alcohol use and sport participation play a significant role in the socialization of most Americans, particularly late adolescents and young adults, alcohol prevention efforts will in most cases have a significant impact on athletes.

Prevention agents within sport may include a variety of individuals such as sport administrators, coaches, health professionals, athletes, organizations, and parents. Since alcohol use is pervasive among athletes and others in the sport world, it is incumbent upon leaders in sport to develop effective prevention strategies to minimize the potential negative impact of alcohol use among athletes. By virtue of their often influential role among their peers, athletes in turn may assist in prevention of alcohol problems among the general population.

HELPING THE PROBLEM DRINKER TO CHANGE

In order to be of assistance to the problem drinker, the helping professional must realize that a significant number of individuals drink alcohol at harm-producing levels, many of these individuals do not receive treatment and are reluctant to seek treatment until late in the development of alcohol problems, and many progress through a self-appraisal or self-change process that contributes to their eventual recovery. Helping professionals may lend the most effective support to problem drinkers by stimulating this self-appraisal process which frequently includes a cognitive evaluation of the pros and cons of drinking.

It has been demonstrated that brief interventions focusing on this cognitive evaluation have been shown to be effective in reducing alcohol consumption and facilitating entry into treatment. It has been hypothesized that these interventions may in effect increase the individual's motivation for change which allows for drinking behavior to be altered with or without formal treatment. This research implies that, given appropriate training in these brief interventions, nonspecialist helping professionals (e.g., physicians, nurses, psychologists, etc.) may provide cost-effective intervention services for problem drinkers. The literature has numerous examples of brief interventions with common elements that have had significant positive impact on drinking behavior directly as well as on treatment seeking. Therefore, helping professionals in a variety of settings (including sport-related settings) may be able to provide effective intervention services for problem drinkers who normally would not avail themselves of treatment.

ALCOHOL TREATMENT AND ATHLETES

Treatment for alcohol problems usually includes a broad range of services with the overall goal to reduce or eliminate the use of alcohol as a factor in associated physical, psychological, and social dysfunctions. Professional help for alcohol abuse takes various forms and intensities. It can be functionally divided into two basic types: (a) pharmacological treatment which includes drugs used to manage withdrawal from alcohol and drugs used in long-term rehabilitation, and (b) psychological treatment which includes behavioral and psychodynamic approaches or multimodal treatments using both approaches. Both pharmacological and psychological treatments are often incorporated together in a treatment program.

Three basic stages of care have been described in the literature including acute intervention, rehabilitation, and maintenance. These stages of care represent a continuum necessary to provide sufficient services for alcohol abusers and dependents experiencing varying levels of severity of alcohol-related problems. Evaluation of the individual's progress is important at entry and exit from each stage of care. If and when relapses occur, reentry into previous stages of care may be necessary.

Since athletes apparently experience similar alcohol abuse problems as the general population, similar treatments will be effective with problem-drinking athletes as they are with problem drinkers from the general population. An important issue to consider, however, is how the sport experience may influence the athlete's treatment seeking and participation. Sport participation may act to either delay or facilitate entry into the acute intervention stage of treatment. Similarly, sport participation may influence the athlete's progression through the rehabilitation and maintenance stages of treatment.

The sport experience may develop skills in the athlete that potentially will have positive influences on treatment outcome. An example of one of these skills is the ability to set and work toward goals. To the extent the athlete comes to treatment with some or all of these skills, treatment may be facilitated. Efforts should be made by alcohol rehabilitation professionals and others to capitalize on these skills by assisting athletes in their transfer from sport to the therapeutic arena. Also, the treatment experience can be used to develop or restore these skills. These mental skills together with an appropriate match to the type and level of treatment needed should enhance treatment outcome for athletes.

While participation in alcohol treatment may be challenging for athletes, particularly as therapeutic demands interfere with the athlete's competitive participation, the rewards of successful outcomes more than compensate for inconveniences that may occur. Successful treatment outcome will not only provide for increased quality of life for the individual, but also will increase the likelihood of a return to former athletic performance levels. Knowledgeable and capable sport professionals who understand how to identify and refer athletes to the appropriate resource for evaluation and treatment set the stage for this favorable result.

FUTURE CONSIDERATIONS

Both alcohol use and sport participation are valued activities in our society and both will likely continue to be a significant part of our way of life. For the reasons discussed previously, the alcohol industry and sport have been strongly linked in the United States. This linkage has been mutually beneficial to both institutions; sport provides a ready-made market with a high percentage of drinkers for the alcohol industry, particularly beer brewers, in exchange for sponsorship and advertising dollars. However, the relationship also has led to some unfortunate side effects. Perhaps the primary untoward side effect is the often implicit message that frequent and heavy drinking are not inconsistent with reaching one's potential in athletic performance. To achieve in sport requires development of mental and physical skills to provide for the greatest likelihood of outstanding performance. While occasional social drinking has not been found to hinder athletic performance, our current understanding of the nature and development of alcohol abuse and dependence does not allow for a precise definition of nonharmful, social drinking.

Therefore, a clear message of what is a safe limit of alcohol consumption for all people is not possible.

Given that alcohol, sport, and their close-knit relationship likely will be a part of the social structure for the foreseeable future, it would behoove us as sport professionals to examine how the alcohol-sport relationship might be altered so that the potential negative consequences of this relationship are minimized. The following suggestions are offered in this regard for sport professionals; however, their application may extend beyond our sport-related roles to subsume our activities as parents, teachers, or community members.

1. Alter the demographics of either the beer drinker, sports fan, or both so that they do not coincide so completely. If this is successful, the beer industry would have less incentive to target their marketing to sports fans. Perhaps the easiest way to accomplish this goal is to encourage broader participation across demographic lines in sport. This would include increasing participation in spectatorship to different age groups, and to both genders. Recently, due to changes in funding for secondary-school and collegiate athletics, female sport participants have increased. Similar movements need to be initiated and continued with older adults and with young children. It is likely that these new sport participants will become spectators as well. The broader the demographic characteristics of sport spectators and participants, the more likely that drinking practices in this population will be heterogeneous and the less likely that alcohol industry advertisers will target sport as a primary marketing population.

2. Encourage the alcohol industry to target other social characteristics than those that are sport related. For instance, moderate and responsible alcohol use may be promoted as consistent with social interaction associated with food consumption. Alcohol consumption in these settings is much less likely to lead to problem-oriented heavy drinking.

3. Reinforce the health aspects of sport for all participants and emphasize the inconsistencies of heavy drinking with the goals of a healthy mind and body. Sport should not be a pastime confined to youth as is the unfortunate circumstance with many Americans. Successfully promoting a lifetime of good health, partly accomplished through physical activity, will in itself be a

major alcohol abuse prevention strategy. To accomplish the goal of lifelong participation in sport, we must do a much better job of encouraging early participation by children and preventing dropout from competitive sport during childhood. On the other end of the developmental spectrum, we must provide legitimate alternatives for adults to continue their participation in sport by providing appropriate facilities, incentives, and instruction.

4. Provide athletes with reasonable alternatives to alcohol use for socializing, stress reduction, and perceived performance enhancement. This goal may be accomplished by appropriate modeling of desired alternatives by coaches and other influential figures (e.g., parents, teachers, administrators), teaching mental skills (e.g., relaxation, imagery, positive self-talk) to enhance performance in sport as well as other life areas, and providing treatment where indicated for appropriate athletes.

Most if not all of the above considerations will not only require changes in the relationship of alcohol to sport but also changes in society's relationship to alcohol. Sport in many ways is a reflection of the values and morals existing in society; how society regards alcohol dictates largely how individuals in sport regard alcohol. Therefore, as a society we must realize the tremendous potential for harm associated with alcohol abuse. Moderation and abstinence should be condoned as reasonable alternatives for alcohol use while heavy drinking and drunkenness should be avoided. Sport professionals may play a major role in stimulating societal changes that reduce the likelihood of negative consequences related to alcohol use. However, to fulfill this role successfully, we must equip ourselves with sufficient knowledge, skills, and motivation to confront alcohol-related issues within sport and our society.

ALCOHOL USE IN SOCIETY

This appendix supplies the reader with a background on alcohol use in society and includes sections on the history of alcohol use, alcohol use in the United States, and a cross-national perspective on alcohol use. Before alcohol use and abuse in sport can be understood, one must be aware of alcohol use in society generally. The first section of this appendix gives the reader a perspective of the vast history of alcohol use worldwide and its role in civilization. The second section on alcohol use in the United States reviews American drinking patterns and how cultural norms affect them. The final section on cross-national perspectives reviews drinking practices in a sample of European countries.

HISTORICAL ROOTS OF ALCOHOL USE

The use of alcoholic beverages is an ancient practice, perhaps dating back to the Paleolithic Age, about 8,000 B.C., when mead was made from honey (Ray & Ksir, 1993, p. 178). Natural fermentation was likely to be the first process used to create beverage alcohol. Brewing beer was probably simultaneous with the discovery of agriculture (because its ingredients are primarily grains) and subsequently spread with the distribution of agriculture throughout the world (Horton, 1991). Distillation, a process to increase the alcohol concentration in beverage, was discovered much later, probably in Arabia around 800 A.D. (Ray & Ksir, 1993, p. 180). The discovery of distillation allowed progressively higher alcohol content beverages to be produced (e.g., whiskey, vodka, gin).

Either by contact with outside cultures or by independent invention, the custom of drinking alcoholic beverages became widely distributed throughout the world. Indeed, as noted by

Horton (1991), the use of alcoholic beverages in various forms was nearly universal. Almost every natural source of sugar has been used to produce a fermented beverage, including a variety of starches for brewing beer. Therefore, the production of alcohol was fairly easy because of the readily available resources to produce it.

The consumption of alcoholic beverages is a custom that has survived many thousands of years in most cultures worldwide. The longevity of this custom has occurred despite competition from other customs, as well as direct opposition to using alcohol because of presumed dangers involved in its use. There have been numerous efforts throughout history to severely restrict or abolish the use of alcohol without success. Therefore, in many cultures (including the United States) there is ambivalence regarding alcohol use. On the one hand, custom has approved of and supported alcohol, and on the other hand, it is a source of fear, which has led to efforts to restrict its use (Horton, 1991).

Alcohol has two properties that underlie its perceived value and have allowed it to sustain itself in the customs of multiple cultures: its anxiety- and tension-reducing qualities and its euphoria-producing qualities. In examining alcohol use patterns in primitive cultures, Horton (1991) suggested that the extent of alcohol consumption in any society directly relates to the amount of anxiety felt by the members of the society, which is proportional to the strength of anxiety-producing factors that exist in a culture. These anxiety-producing factors usually took the form of various environmental stressors such as inadequate or unstable food supply, proximity of enemies, and epidemics. Alcohol also has a sedative quality that reduces social tensions and thus allows for more relaxed social interchange. These desirable psychological effects of alcohol produce a high value for its use and provide a basis for explaining why alcohol use has remained such a common practice in various cultures throughout time. Others have suggested that rather than the anxiety-reducing qualities of alcohol, it is its euphoria-producing qualities that have supported its widespread use. Jellinek (1977) suggested that cultures have incorporated drinking alcohol as a "positive and reinforcing part of their societies, rather than solely in a negative or tension-reducing aspect" (p. 852). Jellinek further explained that in most cultures drinking alcoholic beverages takes on symbolic meaning. For example, the cocktail party signifies equivalent status among those present; teenage drinking is symbolic of desired progression to adulthood; and drinking at a wake symbolizes the mutual support of those in mourning. Drinking in these situations promotes identification among participants and forms symbolic covenants. In addition to the symbolic function of drinking, Jellinek also supported the notion of a utilitarian use for alcohol, the primary one being tension relief. As symbolic reasons for drinking recede and utilitarian reasons take precedence in a culture, there is an increase in individualized drinking. Jellinek suggested that industrialized societies tend to individualize sources of tension and encourage more utilitarian drinking. Therefore, the custom of drinking continues but is in response to needs that are different from societies that promote drinking for symbolic reasons. This utilitarian drinking typically leads to excess alcohol consumption and the need for external controls on alcohol as well as treatment and rehabilitation. Other factors that facilitate the transition from symbolic to utilitarian drinking are mass production of alcohol and preservation techniques, advertising of alcoholic beverages, increased efficiency in the distribution of alcohol, and the influence of parties with vested interests (Jellinek, 1977).

Anthropology and sociology have contributed much to the study of alcohol and society. Perhaps the most important is the understanding of the powerful cultural influences that determine the form alcohol use will take in various societies. An influential book by MacAndrew and Edgerton (1969) suggested that drunken comportment is a product of the expectations and the cultural values regarding drunkenness extant in a particular society rather than alcohol's effects on the brain. The recent widespread emergence of the belief that alcoholism is the product of biopsychosocial factors is a reflection of the importance placed on sociocultural factors in the etiology of alcoholism. Furthermore, the application of the public health model to the development of alcoholism also establishes social and cultural factors as influential in drinking practices and the etiology of alcoholism. An excellent review by Heath (1987; see Heath, 1991, for an abridged version) provides an overview of some of this literature.

ALCOHOL USE IN THE UNITED STATES

Alcohol ranks as the third leading source of calories in the American diet, behind breads and various sweets such as doughnuts and cookies ("Vital Statistics," 1993). This is true despite the fact that many adults abstain from alcohol. Abstinence rates range from 30 percent to 70 percent across the United States. Of those that drink, approximately 21 percent report experiencing social and other consequences from drinking. Therefore, the majority of drinkers (approximately 80 percent) drink without significant alcohol-related problems (see review in USDHHS, 1993).

American Drinking Patterns

Recent analyses of serial surveys done in 1967 and in 1984 suggest that American drinking patterns showed little change over this time (Hilton & Clark, 1991). Changes in beverage preference occurred; for example, more beer and wine than distilled spirits were consumed in 1984 than in 1967. However, when considering total alcohol from all beverage types, the volume of drinks consumed did not change significantly. Few significant differences in drinking patterns occurred; one exception was that the percentage of men reporting abstinence increased slightly. With regard to drinking-related problems, the proportion of survey respondents reporting any of nine problem consequences was unchanged during this 17-year period, but the proportion experiencing dependence-related problems increased. Even though there was an 11.8 percent increase in per capita consumption of alcohol between 1967 and 1984, there apparently was not a concomitant increase in the prevalence of heavy drinking during this time. The authors indicated, however, that the limited sample size might have prevented them from detecting significant differences.

American Cultural Norms

It has been well accepted that cultural norms significantly affect alcohol use. These cultural norms affect the value placed on alcohol use and determine what forms alcohol use will take and how its use will be controlled (Klein, 1991; Lemert, 1991). For example, in a recent survey of alcohol use in the United States, Klein (1991) found that different types of alcohol (wine, beer, spirits, and wine coolers) were both perceived and used differently among Americans. He found that gender and age had significant influences on drinking practices. For instance, he found that women were more knowledgeable about the potential adverse consequences of alcohol, they drank different beverages in different settings than men, and they consumed less alcohol than men. In addition, men and women differed in terms of emotional states that precipitated drinking. With regard to age effects, young drinkers drank in response to a greater number of emotional states, and older drinkers drank whenever they wanted to and were less responsive to affective conditions at the time. Klein concluded from his study that cultural factors play major roles in how various alcoholic beverages are used in society as well as how male and female and young and old drinkers choose to use alcohol.

Because the United States is a multiethnic and multiracial nation, these variables have been examined regarding their influence on alcohol use. Numerous studies have indicated that ethnic and racial differences in alcohol use exist, but the literature has reported few viable explanations for these variations (Cheung, 1990–91). Complicating the issue is that significant heterogeneity in drinking patterns has been found within minority groups (Lex, 1987). It appears that racial-ethnic groupings may not be as meaningful for alcohol use patterns as consumption level groupings. Indeed, reasons for drinking have varied much more across groups with different alcohol consumption levels, independent of ethnicity, than across racial-ethnic groups (Johnson, Schwitters, Wilson, Nagoshi, & McClearn, 1985).

Some authors (Cheung, 1990–1991; Heath, 1991) have suggested that the reason we can't explain ethnic variations in alcohol use is that most studies have not properly conceptualized and measured the variable of ethnicity. Factors to consider when investigating the ethnicity-alcohol use relationship include the degree to which individuals identify with their ethnic origin, how they have incorporated into the mainstream culture and the problems resulting from this adaptation, generational status and age at immigration (if they are not native born), and their involvement in their ethnic community. With these variables considered, perhaps we can understand the impact of ethnic origin on alcohol use.

In addition to the individual variables described (gender, age, ethnicity), environmental variables, such as the setting in which drinking takes place, have strong effects on drinking practices. Learning to drink in America is a highly social activity and is predominantly influenced by family and peers (White, Bates, & Johnson, 1991). Initiation of drinking most often occurs within a family and is largely determined by parental guidance and modeling. As adolescence progresses, however, peers become a strong influence on alcohol and drug use. In fact, the drinking and drug use practices of friends have consistently shown strong relationships to the onset and patterning of alcohol and drug use among adolescents (Kandel, 1980). Orcutt (1991) found that the presence of close friends significantly affected the volume of alcohol adolescent heavy drinkers consumed. In addition, he found that the presence of friends also altered the subjective effects of alcohol, therefore enhancing the intoxicating effects of relatively few drinks. Adult alcohol consumption also is influenced by contextual variables such as the size of drinking groups and consumption rate of drinking partners (Single, 1987). These environmental variables may hold promise to explain drinking patterns including consumption, intoxication, and related alcohol problems.

CROSS-NATIONAL PERSPECTIVE ON ALCOHOL USE

Although a detailed discussion of alcohol use patterns in other countries is beyond the scope of this book, it is important to note that alcohol use is a worldwide phenomenon and its form varies in different countries depending on cultural customs that influence its use. For example, in Sweden, where alcohol use is an accepted social custom, there are strict laws to discourage drinking and driving. Sweden has a long history of punishment for drinking and driving, including imprisonment, and recent legislation has lowered the legal level of blood alcohol content (BAC) of drivers to .02. Although there is disagreement among Swedes regarding the need for this strict law, Havard (1990) suggests that young novice drivers, who are overrepresented in alcohol-related automobile accidents, may benefit.

Recent studies on alcohol use among adolescents in Britain suggest that, as in the United States, there is concern over the apparent increase in heavy drinking by young people (Sharp & Lowe, 1989). The comments by Sharp and Lowe regarding alcohol use by British adolescents are strikingly similar to American authors on the same subject. There is suggestion of acceptance that adolescents will experiment with alcohol, because survey data indicate such is the case. The authors have suggested, however, that to encourage sensible drinking practices it is important for research to answer the question of why adolescents drink and what meaning drinking has for this population.

In France during the last 15 years, average alcohol consumption has moderated and even started to decrease (d'Houtaud, Adriaanse, & Field, 1989). Just as in the United States, it appears that many young male drinkers in France consume large quantities of alcohol and are disproportionately represented in traffic accidents related to alcohol (Delaunay, Balkau, & Papoz, 1991). In 1990, as part of a national health promotion program, new legislation was introduced in France that bans the advertising of alcoholic beverages with few exceptions (Comiti, 1990). D'Houtaud et al. indicated that the data needed to assess the changes in alcohol consumption in France, as well as the potential reasons for changes, are largely nonexistent. Factors potentially associated with change in drinking behaviors have been hypothesized, but the overall model has yet to be explored (d'Houtaud et al.)

A recent study on alcohol consumption trends in Spain, Portugal, France, and Italy indicated that overall consumption levels have declined in Spain, France, and Italy and wine consumption has declined in all four countries (Pyorala, 1990). Beer (a lower alcohol content beverage) has evidently replaced wine as the most commonly consumed alcoholic beverage in Spain, Portugal, and Italy. In France, the decline in wine consumption has not been replaced by use of another alcoholic beverage. In Spain (Alvarez, Queipo, Del Rio, & Garcia, 1991) and Italy (Monarca et al., 1991) there have been reports of increased concern about drunkenness among young people. In Spain, beer has become the preferred drink among the young, with more extensive consumption occurring on weekends and by males (Alvarez, 1991; Alvarez et al., 1991).

Although cross-cultural comparisons have been made about drinking practices, these studies have been descriptive. Attempts to construct theory to account for cultural differences in drinking practices have met with many problems, as noted by Hartka and Fillmore (1989). This lack of theory is likely to change because of growing interest in replicating research findings across diverse cultures and the increasing availability of data across cultures, as well as methodologies to handle this data. An excellent example of increased cooperation across national boundaries is the recent effort to collect epidemiological data on alcoholism across cultural regions in North America, Europe, and Asia (Helzer & Canino, 1992). This study is unique in that it incorporates standard measurement devices that were translated and adapted for use in each of the cultures that were measured. In addition, the authors took a multidisciplinary approach to the study of alcoholism, yielding results that have significantly greater explanatory value than mere prevalence estimates. Although the focus of this project was on alcoholism, there is sufficient description of drinking practices in each of the cultural groups to draw some conclusions regarding the relationships between drinking practices and the incidence of alcoholism.

RESOURCES

ALCOHOL ABUSE AND DEPENDENCE

The following organizations provide information regarding alcohol abuse and dependence and their treatment.

Hazelden
P.O. Box 11
Center City, MN 55012-0011
800-257-7800 Information Center
800-328-9000 Educational Materials

Hazelden provides rehabilitation, education, and professional services for chemical dependency and related addictive disorders.

National Clearinghouse for Alcohol and Drug Information
    (NCADI)
P.O. Box 2345
Rockville, MD 20847-2345
800-729-6686

NCADI is a distributor of information from federal organizations involved in alcohol and drug abuse education, prevention, and treatment efforts. These include the Center for Substance Abuse Prevention, Center for Substance Abuse Treatment, National Institute on Alcohol Abuse and Alcoholism, and National Institute on Drug Abuse.

Rutgers Center of Alcohol Studies
Smithers Hall, Busch Campus
Piscataway, NJ 08855-0969
908-445-4442

The Rutgers Center maintains a comprehensive collection of books, periodicals, dissertations, reports, and other material relat-

ing to alcohol studies. Reference, circulation, interlibrary loan, and document delivery services are available.

ALCOHOL ABUSE PREVENTION PROGRAMS

The following resources provide practical information on developing and implementing alcohol and drug abuse prevention programs within sport.

Secondary School Level

Deighan, W.P., et al. (1986). *Team up for drug prevention with America's young athletes.* Washington, DC: Drug Enforcement Administration. (ERIC Document Reproduction Service No. ED 274 934)

Division of Alcohol and Drug Education Services. Bureau of Instruction in Maine. (1988). *Guidelines for assisting athletes with alcohol and other drug problems.* Reston, VA: National Association for Sport and Physical Education. (Reproduced with permission in 1988 and available through the National Association for Sport and Physical Education, 1900 Association Drive, Reston, VA 22091)

Drug Enforcement Agency. (1986). *For coaches only: How to start a drug prevention program.* Washington, DC: Author. (ERIC Document Reproduction Service No. ED 274 933)

Svendsen, R., Griffin, T., & McIntyre, D.E. (Eds.) (1984). *Chemical health: School athletics and fine arts activities.* Center City, MN: Hazelden Foundation.

Collegiate and Professional Level

Grossman, S.J., & Gieck, J. (1992). A model alcohol and other drug peer education program for student athletes. *Journal of Sport Rehabilitation, 1,* 337–349.

Grossman, S.J., Gieck, J., Freedman, A., & Fang, W.L. (1993). The athletic prevention programming and leadership education (APPLE) model: Developing substance abuse prevention programs. *Journal of Athletic Training, 28,* 137–138, 140, 142, 144.

Techniques for Effective Alcohol Management (TEAM). For information regarding this coalition of private and public agencies involved in alcohol prevention contact Global Exchange, 7910 Woodmont Avenue, Suite 400, Bethesda, MD 20814-3015. 301-656-3100

Tricker, R., & Cook, D. (1993). (Eds.) *Athletes at risk: Drugs and sport.* Dubuque, IA: Brown & Benchmark.

Wadler, G.I., & Hainline, B. (1989). *Drugs and the athlete.* Philadelphia: F.A. Davis. This book contains appendixes with alcohol and drug use policies of major sport organizations.

QUESTIONS FOR DISCUSSION

Given the widespread use of alcohol and the serious consequences of its abuse, it is likely that most of us will be negatively affected, in one way or another, by our own or others' intemperate alcohol use. Because I and many of the readers of this book are in helping professions related to the well-being of athletes, it is important that we understand the risks associated with alcohol. Although part of this understanding is based on knowledge of alcohol and addiction, perhaps a greater understanding will come from self-exploration regarding personal attitudes about alcohol and from exploring ways our society may shape the alcohol use patterns of the general population and the sport community. It is in hopes of stimulating this understanding that I pose the following questions for your consideration.

CHAPTER 1

1. Because alcohol is pervasive across many cultures, it is important for individuals to formulate some ideas or philosophy regarding its use. What is your philosophy and how does it interact with those individuals most important to you and with your primary culture's views?

2. Given that some percentage of a population will experience problems related to alcohol use, what is society's obligation or role in assisting these individuals to resolve their alcohol-related problems? Can and should society play a role in preventing alcohol-related problems? Who should act as treatment or prevention agents and in what roles?

3. Alcohol dependence may have biological, psychological, and social causes that vary in importance with the individual. After having read this chapter, what are your beliefs about the causes of alcohol dependence?

CHAPTER 2

1. Alcohol and sport have a long history of association in the United States. What are your thoughts about this association? Is it a mutually enhancing relationship? Are there characteristics of the relationship that are exploitative or abusive?

2. A reasonable conclusion from this chapter is that athletes' alcohol use reflects alcohol use in the general population from which they originate. Is this a reasonable expectation for athletes' drinking habits or should they be expected to demonstrate other alcohol use patterns, particularly if heavy drinking is common in their culture? What about this issue as it applies to sport professionals, such as coaches, administrators, and health professionals?

3. Alcohol use has been a common ingredient in the tragedies associated with fan violence. Administrators have taken measures to decrease the negative impact of alcohol on sport events as described in the chapter. If given the opportunity, what measures might you recommend to curtail the potential negative consequences of alcohol use at sport events?

CHAPTER 3

1. Given our present understanding of alcohol's effects on sport performance, what message might you carry to athletes regarding alcohol use?

2 When providing treatment services, the health professional will consider the risk to benefit ratio of the treatment before proceeding. Applying this principle to drinking alcohol, what risk to benefit ratio would you give to alcohol? What factors might alter this ratio?

CHAPTER 4

1. Athletes and sport professionals have risk factors for alcohol abuse and dependence pertaining to their sport and professional activities. What steps could we take to reduce the influence of these risk factors and how might we implement them?

2. It is frequently difficult for problem drinkers to realize the seriousness of their drinking and to seek appropriate treatment. As helping professionals, it is important to remove potential bar-

riers that deter individuals from receiving treatment. In the case of alcohol-abusing athletes and sport professionals, what are the potential barriers to treatment and how might they be removed?

CHAPTER 5

1. As described in this chapter, both alcohol use and sport participation play a role in the socialization of most youth in the United States. Given this, how might we design alcohol prevention programs for athletes? Should these prevention programs be similar to or different from prevention programs for the general population? If we design programs for athletes differently, what aspects of the programs should we alter?

2. High-profile athletes who have experienced problems with alcohol and drugs often have been spokespersons for alcohol and drug abuse prevention efforts. What are your views about this practice? How do you think their history of alcohol and drug abuse affects their ability to have positive impact on the drinking practices of youth?

3. This chapter contains suggestions for alcohol abuse prevention programs for athletes. Are there other potential components that you think are essential for success in preventing alcohol abuse and dependence among athletes? Are there components listed in this chapter that you believe are unnecessary for successful prevention programs?

CHAPTER 6

1. This chapter presented information regarding the stages and processes that many alcohol abusers or dependents progress through during their recovery. Does this model of change fit with your ideas about how individuals recover from alcohol abuse or dependence? If not, how do your ideas differ?

2. This chapter discussed brief interventions that have been effective in altering problem drinking. It was suggested that helping professionals may be able to provide these brief interventions effectively and therefore use them with problem drinkers who they see in their professional work settings. What do you think your comfort level would be if, after necessary training, you would provide these brief interventions to athletes

in your work setting? Are there factors in your professional or personal history that might interfere with your ability to effectively intervene with problem-drinking athletes?

CHAPTER 7

1. As described in this chapter, alcohol treatment comes in a variety of modalities, settings, and intensities. What is your understanding of alcohol treatment and how might you increase your understanding so you could provide the best guidance for athletes needing this type of treatment?

2. Reviewed in this chapter are six conclusions about alcohol treatment drawn from the literature by Miller (1990). How do these conclusions fit with your notions about alcohol treatment, and how do they affect the manner in which you might handle an athlete who is a candidate for alcohol treatment?

3. This chapter reviews ways in which sport participation may either delay or facilitate entry and completion of alcohol treatment. As a helping professional involved in referring and possibly following an athlete after alcohol treatment, how might you act to facilitate the treatment process and enable the athlete to successfully negotiate the stages of treatment?

REFERENCES

Adrian, M., Layne, N., & Williams, R.T. (1990–1991). Estimating the effect of Native Indian population on county alcohol consumption: The example of Ontario. *The International Journal of the Addictions, 25,* 731–765.

Alcohol, infectious diseases, and immunity. (1992). *Alcohol Health & Research World, 16*(1).

Alcohol-related incidents down in major league ballparks. (1991, October). *The Major League Baseball Newsletter, 5,* 4, 9.

Alterman, A.I., & Tarter, R.E. (1983). The transmission of psychological vulnerability: Implications for alcoholism etiology. *The Journal of Nervous and Mental Disease, 171,* 147–154.

Alvarez, F.J. (1991). Trends in alcohol consumption in Spain. [Letter to the editor.] *British Journal of Addiction, 86,* 104–105.

Alvarez, F.J., Queipo, D., Del Rio, M.C., & Garcia, M.C. (1991). Alcohol consumption in young adults in the rural communities of Spain. *Alcohol & Alcoholism, 26,* 93–101.

American College of Sports Medicine. (1982). The use of alcohol in sports. *Medicine and Science in Sports and Exercise, 14,* ix–xi.

American Psychiatric Association. (1994). *Diagnostic and statistical manual of mental disorders* (4th ed.). Washington, DC: Author.

Amodeo, M., & Kurtz, N. (1990). Cognitive processes and abstinence in a treated alcoholic population. *The International Journal of the Addictions, 25,* 983–1009.

Amusa, L.O., & Muoboghare, P.A. (1986). The effect of three dosages of alcohol on physical performance. *Snipes Journal* (Patiala, India), *9* (2), 46–53.

Anderson, P. (1993). Management of alcohol problems: The role of the general practitioner. *Alcohol & Alcoholism, 28,* 263–272.

Anderson, W.A., Albrecht, R.R., McKeag, D.B., Hough, D.O., & McGrew, C.A. (1991). A national survey of alcohol and drug use by college athletes. *The Physician and Sports Medicine, 19* (2), 91–94, 96–98, 101–102, 104.

Andreasson, S., Allebeck, P., & Brandt, L. (1993). Predictors of alcoholism in young Swedish men. *American Journal of Public Health, 83,* 845–850.

Anshel, M.H. (1991). Cognitive-behavioral strategies for combating drug abuse in sport: Implications for coaches and sport psychology consultants. *The Sport Psychologist, 5,* 152–166.

Ardolino, F. (1991). Dives, dark clubhouses, deceptive dreamscapes, and clean, well-lighted places in sports literature and film. *Aethlon, 8 (2),* 35–54.

Arkansas court finds school's anti-alcohol policy unenforceable. (1989). *Sports and the Courts, 10*(3), 3–4.

Armor, D.J., Polich, J.M., & Stambul, H.B. (1978). *Alcoholism and treatment.* New York: John Wiley.

Atkin, C.K. (1987). Alcoholic-beverage advertising: Its content and impact. In N.K. Mello (Series Eds.) & H.D. Holder (Vol. Ed.) *Advances in substance abuse: behavioral and biological research: Supplement 1: Control issues in alcohol abuse prevention: Strategies for states and communities* (pp. 267–287). Greenwich, CT: JAI Press.

Atkinson, R.M. (1988). Alcoholism in the elderly population [Editorial]. *Mayo Clinic Proceedings, 63,* 825–829.

Atkinson, R.M., Tolson, R.L., & Turner, J.A. (1990). Late versus early onset problem drinking in older men. *Alcoholism: Clinical and Experimental Research, 14,* 574–579.

Babor, T.F., Hofmann, M., DelBoca, F.K., Hasselbrock, V., Meyer, R.E., Dolinsky, Z.S., & Rounsaville, B. (1992). Types of alcoholics, I: Evidence for an empirically derived typology based on indicators of vulnerability and severity. *Archives of General Psychiatry, 49,* 599–608.

Babor, T.F., Kranzler, H.R., & Kadden, R.M. (1986). Issues in the diagnosis of alcoholism: Implications for a reformulation. *Progress in Neuro-Psychopharmacology & Biological Psychiatry, 10,* 113–128.

Bakker, R. (1992). *The coach's role in alcohol/drug prevention* (Clearinghouse Fact Sheet). Piscataway, NJ: Rutgers University, Center of Alcohol Studies.

Baylor, A.M., Layne, C.S., Mayfield, R.D., Osborne, L., & Spirduso, W.W. (1989). Effect of ethanol on human fractionated response times. *Drug and Alcohol Dependence, 23,* 31–40.

Bien, T.H., Miller, W.R., & Tonigan, J.S. (1993). Brief interventions for alcohol problems: A review. *Addiction, 88,* 315–336.

Bissell, L., & Skorina, J.K. (1987). One hundred alcoholic women in medicine: An interview study. *JAMA, 257,* 2939–2944.

Blane, H.T. (1988). Prevention issues with children of alcoholics. *British Journal of Addiction, 83,* 793–798.

Blane, H.T., & Leonard, K.E. (Eds.) (1987). *Psychological theories of drinking and alcoholism.* New York: Guilford Press.

Blankfield, A. (1986). Psychiatric symptoms in alcohol dependence: Diagnostic and treatment implications. *Journal of Substance Abuse Treatment, 3,* 275–278.

Blose, J.O., & Holder, H.D. (1991). The utilization of medical care by treated alcoholics: Longitudinal patterns by age, gender, and type of care. *Journal of Substance Abuse, 3,* 13–27.

Blot, W.J., McLaughlin, J.K., Winn, D.M., Austin, D.F., Greenberg, R.S., Preston-Martin, S., Bernstein, L., Schoenberg, J.B., Stemhagen, A., & Fraumeni, J.F. (1988). Smoking and drinking in relation to oral pharyngeal cancer. *Cancer Research, 48,* 3282–3287.

Blum, K. (1984). *Handbook of abusable drugs*. New York: Gardner Press.

Bond, V., Franks, B.D., & Howley, E.T. (1984). Alcohol, cardiorespiratory function and work performance. *British Journal of Sports Medicine, 18,* 203–206.

Bond, V., Gresham, K.E., Balkissoon, B., & Clearwater, H.E. (1984). Effects of small and moderate doses of alcohol on peak torque and average torque in an isokinetic contraction. *Scandinavian Journal of Sports Science, 6* (1), 1–5.

Borg, G., Domserius, M., & Kaijser, L. (1990). Effect of alcohol on perceived exertion in relation to heart rate and blood lactate. *European Journal of Applied Physiology and Occupational Physiology, 60,* 382–384.

Bowden, S.C. (1990). Separating cognitive impairment in neurologically asymptomatic alcoholism from Wenicke-Korsakoff syndrome: Is the neuropsychological distinction justified? *Psychological Bulletin 107,* 355–366.

Brewer, C. (1993). Invited review: Recent developments in disulfiram treatment. *Alcohol & Alcoholism, 28,* 383–395.

Brownell, K.D., Marlatt, G.A., Lichtenstein, E., & Wilson, G.T. (1986). Understanding and preventing relapse. *American Psychologist, 41,* 765–782.

Buchanan, D.R., & Lev, J. (1989). *Beer and fast cars: How brewers target blue-collar youth through motor sport sponsorships.* Washington, DC: AAA Foundation for Traffic Safety.

Bucholz, K.K., Homan, S.M., & Helzer, J.E. (1992). When do alcoholics first discuss drinking problems? *Journal of Studies on Alcohol, 53,* 582–589.

Byrd, L. (1991a, May 14). Alcohol sport's uncontrolled substance. *The Houston Post,* pp. B1, B8.

Byrd, L. (1991b, May 15). Pressure enough to drive stars to drink. *The Houston Post,* pp. C1, C10.

Caetano, R. (1987). Acculturation and drinking patterns among U.S. Hispanics. *British Journal of Addiction, 82,* 789–799.

Caetano, R. (1989). Drinking patterns and alcohol problems in a national sample of U.S. Hispanics. In D.L. Spiegler, D.A. Tate, S.S. Aitken, & C.M. Christian (Eds.), *Alcohol use among U.S. ethnic minorities: Proceedings of a conference on the epidemiology of alcohol use and abuse among ethnic minority groups* (Research Monograph No. 18) (pp. 147–162). Rockford, MD: National Institute on Alcohol Abuse and Alcoholism.

Cahalan, D. (1988). Foreword. In C.D. Chaudron & D.A. Wilkinson (Eds.), *Theories on alcoholism* (pp. xix–xxv). Toronto, Canada: Addiction Research Foundation.

Campbell, K.E., Zobeck, T.S., Bertolucci, D. (1995). Trends in alcohol-related fatal traffic crashes, United States: 1977–1993 (Surveillance Report #34). Bethesda, MD: National Institute on Alcohol Abuse and Alcoholism.

Carr, C.N., Kennedy, S.R., & Dimick, K.M. (1990). Alcohol use among high school athletes: A comparison of alcohol use and intoxication in male and female high school athletes and non-athletes. *Journal of Alcohol and Drug Education, 36* (1), 39–43.

Chappell, J.N. (1987). Drug use and abuse in the athlete. In J.R. May & M.J. Asken (Eds.), *Sport psychology: The psychological health of the athlete* (pp. 187–211). New York: PMA.

Cherpitel, C.J. (1991). Drinking patterns and problems among primary care patients: A comparison with the general population. *Alcohol & Alcoholism, 26,* 627–633.

Cheung, Y.W. (1990–91). Ethnicity and alcohol/drug use revisited: A framework for future research. *The International Journal of the Addictions, 25,* 581–605.

Coleman, E. (1989, October/November). The news on booze: Alcohol's unsettling effect on cycling performance. *Bicycling, 30,* 70–71.

Collins, W.E. (1980). Performance effects of alcohol intoxication and hangover at ground level and at simulated altitude. *Aviation, Space, and Environmental Medicine, 51,* 327–335.

Comiti, V.P. (1990). The advertising of alcohol in France. *World Health Forum, 11,* 242–245.

Cook, R.F., & Roehl, J.A. (1993). National evaluation of the community partnership program: Preliminary findings. In R.C. Davis, A.J. Lurigio, & D.P. Rosenbaum (Eds.), *Drugs and the community: Involving community residents in combatting the sale of illegal drugs* (pp. 225–248). Springfield, IL: Charles C. Thomas.

Coopersmith, S. (1964). The effects of alcohol on reaction to affective stimuli. *Quarterly Journal of Studies on Alcohol, 25,* 459–475.

Corcoran, J.P., & Feltz, D.L. (1993). Evaluation of chemical health education for high school athletic coaches. *The Sport Psychologist, 7,* 298–308.

Corry, J.M., & Cimbolic, P. (1985). *Drugs: Facts, alternatives, decisions.* Belmont, CA: Wadsworth.

Crawford, S. (1977). Sport and alcohol. *The New Zealand Journal of Health, Physical Education and Recreation, 10* (3), 76–79, 81–82.

Crosby, L.R., & Bissell, L. (1989). *To care enough: Intervention with chemically dependent colleagues: A guide for healthcare and other professionals.* Minneapolis, MN: Johnson Institute.

Danish, S.J., & D'Augelli, A.R. (1983). *Helping skills II: Life development intervention: Trainee's workbook.* New York: Human Sciences.

Danish, S.J., Petitpas, A.J., & Hale, B.D. (1990). Sport as a context for developing competence. In T.P. Gullotta, G.R. Adams, & R. Montemayor (Series & Vol. Eds.), *Advances in adolescent development: An annual book series: Vol. 3. Developing social competency in adolescence* (pp. 169–194). Newbury Park, CA. Sage.

DeBakey, S.F., Stinson, F.S., Grant, B.F., & Dufour, M.C. (1995). *Liver cirrhosis mortality in the United States, 1970–1992* (Surveillance Report No. 25). Bethesda, MD: National Institute on Alcohol Abuse and Alcoholism.

Delaunay, C., Balkau, B., Papoz, L. (1991). Frequency of alcoholisation among young people injured in accidents in France. *Alcohol & Alcoholism, 26,* 391–397.

d'Houtaud, A., Adriaanse, H., & Field, M.G. (1989). Alcohol consumption in France: Production, consumption, morbidity and mortality, prevention and education in the last three decades. *Advances in Alcohol and Substance Abuse, 8* (1), 19–44.

Dickinson, A.L. (1979, March). Medical advice. *Nordic World, 7,* 62–63.

Drug Enforcement Administration. (1986). *For coaches only: How to start a drug prevention program.* Washington, DC: Author. (ERIC Document Reproduction Service No. ED 274 933).

Drug-free Schools and Communities Act of 1986, 20 U.S.C.A.§3171 *et seq.* (West 1990 & Supp. 1996)

Drug-free Workplace Act of 1988, 41 U.S.C.A.§701 *et seq.* (West Supp. 1996)

Dryfoos, J.G. (1990). *Adolescents at risk: Prevalence and prevention.* New York: Oxford University Press.

Dube, C.E., Goldstein, M.G., Lewis, D.C., Cyr, M.G., & Zwick, W.R. (1989). Project ADEPT: The development process for a competency-based alcohol and drug curriculum for primary care physicians. *Substance Abuse, 10* (1), 5–15.

Eckardt, M.J., & Martin, P.R. (1986). Clinical assessment of cognition in alcoholism. *Alcoholism: Clinical and experimental research, 10,* 123–127.

Edwards, G., & Gross, M.M. (1976). Alcohol dependence: Provisional description of a clinical syndrome. *British Medical Journal, 1,* 1058–1061.

Edwards, H. (1973). *Sociology of sport.* Homewood, IL: Dorsey Press.

Eller, C. (1988, March/April). Role models reach youth. *Alcoholism and Addiction, 8,* 46.

Evans, M., Weinberg, R., & Jackson, A. (1992). Psychological factors related to drug use in college athletes. *The Sport Psychologist, 6,* 24–41.

Fe Caces, M., Stinson, F.S., & Dufour, M.C. (1995). *Trends in alcohol-related morbidity among short-stay community hospital discharges, United States, 1979–1993* (Surveillance Report No. 36). Bethesda, MD: National Institute on Alcohol Abuse and Alcoholism.

Fillmore, K.M. (1987). Prevalence, incidence, and chronicity of drinking patterns and problems among men as a function of age: A longitudinal and cohort analysis. *British Journal of Addiction, 82,* 77–83.

Fimrite, R. (1990, September 17). 1 pitch at a time: With the same resolve that governs his life as a recovering alcoholic, Bob Welch has pitched his way to a Cy Young-caliber season. *Sports Illustrated, 73,* 58–60, 63.

Flaherty, J.A., & Richman, J.A. (1993). Substance use and addiction among medical students, residents, and physicians. *Psychiatric Clinics of North America, 16* (1), 189–197.

Frey, R.D. (1973). *Selected socio-psychological characteristics of hockey, rugby, and soccer players.* Unpublished master's thesis, California State University, San Diego.

Friedman, H. (1992). Alcohol, arrhythmia, and sudden death. *Alcohol, Health and Research World, 16,* 87–92.

Funkhouser, J.E., & Denniston, R.W. (1992). Historical perspective. In M.A. Jansen, S. Becker, M. Klitzner, & K. Stewart (Eds.), *A promising future: Alcohol and other drug problem prevention services improvement* (OSAP Prevention Monograph No. 10) (pp. 5–15). Rockville, MD: Office for Substance Abuse Prevention.

Funkhouser, J.E., Goplerud, E.N., & Bass, R.O. (1992). Current status of prevention strategies. In M.A. Jansen, S. Becker, M. Klitzner, & K. Stewart (Eds.), *A promising future: Alcohol and other drug problem prevention services improvement* (OSAP Prevention Monograph No. 10) (pp. 17–82). Rockville, MD: Office for Substance Abuse Prevention.

Gallmeier, C.P. (1988). Juicing, burning, and tooting: Observing drug use among professional hockey players. *Arena Review, 12* (1), 1–12.

Goldman, M.S. (1986). Neuropsychological recovery in alcoholics: Endogenous and exogenous processes. *Alcoholism: Clinical and Experimental Research, 10,* 136–144.

Goldman, M.S. (1987). The role of time and practice in recovery of function in alcoholics. In O.A. Parsons, N. Butters, & P.E. Nathan (Eds.), *Neuropsychology of alcoholism: Implications for diagnosis and treatment* (pp. 291–321). New York: Guilford Press.

Good, P. (1985). Chemical awareness: Why do young athletes abuse alcohol and drugs? *Interscholastic Athletic Administration, 12* (1), 8–9, 11–13, 15.

Goodwin, D.W. (1992). Alcohol: Clinical aspects. In J.H. Lowinson, P. Ruiz, R.B. Millman, & J.G. Langrod (Eds.), *Substance abuse: A comprehensive textbook* (2nd ed.) (pp. 144–151). Baltimore: Williams & Wilkins.

Gould, R.A., & Clum, G.A. (1993). A meta-analysis of self-help treatment approaches. *Clinical Psychology Review, 13,* 169–186.

Grant, B.F., DeBakey, S., & Zobeck, T.S. (1991). *Liver cirrhosis mortality in the United States, 1973–1988* (Surveillance Report No. 18). Rockville, MD: National Institute on Alcohol Abuse & Alcoholism.

Grant, B.F., Harford, T.C., Chou, P., Pickering, R., Dawson, D.A., Stinson, F.S., & Noble, J. (1991). Prevalence of DSM-III-R alcohol abuse and dependence: United States, 1988. *Alcohol, Health & Research World, 15,* 91–96.

Green, E.K., Burke, K.L. Nix, C.L., Lambrecht, K.W., & Mason, D.C. (1995). Psychological factors associated with alcohol use by high school athletes. *Journal of Sport Behavior, 18,* 195–208.

Green, P. (1989). The chemically dependent nurse. *Nursing Clinics of North America, 24* (1), 81–94.

Greenfield, T.K. (1995). *Who drinks most of the alcohol in the U.S.? The policy implications.* Paper presented at the 39th International Institute on the Prevention and Treatment of Alcoholism, International Council on Alcohol and Alcoholism, Trieste, Italy.

Greising, D. (1993, April 12). Baseball's owners are finally taking a whack at the ball. *Business Week, 66–69.*

Griffin, T., & Newman, M. (1989). Athletics and chemical use: The role of student athletes as peer leaders. In R.B. Waahlberg (Ed.), *Proceedings of the 35th International Congress on Alcoholism and Drug Dependence: Volume II. Prevention and control/realities and aspirations* (pp. 166–172). Oslo, Norway: National Directorate for the Prevention of Alcohol and Drug Problems.

Hansen, W.B. (1992). School-based substance abuse prevention: A review of the state of the art in curriculum, 1980–1990. *Health Education Research, 7,* 403–430.

Hansen, W.B. (1993). School-based alcohol prevention programs. *Alcohol Health & Research World, 17,* 54–60.

Harding, W.M., Apsler, R., & Goldfein, J. (1988). *The assessment of ride service programs as an alcohol countermeasure* (NHTSA Final Report No. DOT HS-807-290). Washington, DC: National Highway Traffic Safety Administration. (NTIS No. PB88-240726)

Hartka, E., & Fillmore, K.M. (1989). Cross-cultural and cross-temporal explanations of drinking behavior: Contributions from epidemiology, life-span development psychology and the sociology of aging. *British Journal of Addiction, 84,* 1409–1417.

Harvey, C. (1991, July/August). Safe sips: Athletics and alcohol should be paired with care. *Women's Sport and Fitness, 13,* 16, 18.

Havard, J. (1990). Sweden lowers blood alcohol limit for drivers. *British Medical Journal, 300,* 1482.

Hayashida, M., Alterman, A.I., McLellan, A.T., O'Brien, C.P., Purtill, J.J., Volpicelli, J.R., Raphaelson, A.H., & Hall, C.P. (1989). Comparative effectiveness and costs of inpatient and outpatient detoxification of patients with mild-to-moderate alcohol withdrawal syndrome. *The New England Journal of Medicine, 320,* 358–365.

Hayes, R.W., & Tevis, B.W. (1977). A comparison of attitudes and behavior of high school athletes and non-athletes with respect to alcohol use and abuse. *Journal of Alcohol and Drug Education, 23* (1), 20–28.

Heath, D.B. (1987). Anthropology and alcohol studies: Current issues. In B.J. Siegel, A.R. Beals, & S.A. Tyler (Eds.), *Annual review of anthropology: Vol. 16* (pp. 99–120). Palo Alto, CA: Annual Reviews.

Heath, D.B. (1988). Emerging anthropological theory and models of alcohol use and alcoholism. In C.D. Chaudron & D.A. Wilkinson (Eds.), *Theories on alcoholism* (pp. 353–410). Toronto: Addiction Research Foundation.

Heath, D.B. (1991). Alcohol studies and anthropology. In D.J. Pittman & H.R. White (Eds.), *Society, culture, and drinking patterns reexamined* (pp. 87–108). New Brunswick, NJ: Rutgers Center of Alcohol Studies.

Heikkonen, E. (1989). *Endocrine and metabolic changes induced by alcohol and physical exercise in healthy males.* Helsinki, Finland: Turku.

Heitzinger & Associates. (1986). *1981–1986 Data collection and analysis: High school, college, professional athletes alcohol/drug survey.* Madison, WI: Author.

Helzer, J.E., & Canino, G.J. (Eds.) (1992). *Alcoholism in North America, Europe, and Asia.* New York: Oxford University Press.

Helzer, J.E., & Pryzbeck, T.R. (1988). The co-occurrence of alcoholism with other psychiatric disorders in the general population and its impact on treatment. *Journal of Studies on Alcohol, 49,* 219–224.

Herd, D. (1987). Rethinking black drinking [Editorial]. *British Journal of Addiction, 82,* 219–223.

Herd, D. (1989). The epidemiology of drinking patterns and alcohol-related problems among U.S. blacks. In D. Spiegler, D. Tate, S. Aitken, & C. Christian (Eds.), *Alcohol use among U.S. ethnic minorities: Proceedings of a conference on the epidemiology of alcohol use and abuse among ethnic minority groups* (Research Monograph No. 18, pp. 3–50). Rockville, MD: National Institute on Alcohol Abuse and Alcoholism.

Hester, R.K., & Miller, W.R. (Eds.) (1989). *Handbook of alcoholism treatment approaches: Effective alternatives.* New York: Pergamon Press.

Hiestand, M. (1993, July 23). Targeting demographics: "Wave of future." *USA Today,* p. 10c.

Hilton, M.E. (1991a). The demographic distribution of drinking problems in 1984. In W.B. Clark & M.E. Hilton (Eds.), *Alcohol in America: Drinking practices and problems* (pp. 87– 101). Albany, NY: State University of New York Press.

Hilton, M.E. (1991b). A note on measuring drinking problems in the 1984 national alcohol survey. In W.B. Clark & M.E. Hilton (Eds.), *Alcohol in America: Drinking practices and problems* (pp. 51–70). Albany, NY: State University of New York Press.

Hilton, M.E., & Clark, W.B. (1987). Changes in American drinking patterns and problems, 1967–1984. *Journal of Studies on Alcohol, 48,* 515–522.

Hilton, M.E., & Clark, W.B. (1991). Changes in American drinking patterns and problems, 1967–1984. In D.J. Pittman & H.R. White (Eds.), *Society, culture, and drinking patterns reexamined* (pp. 157–172). New Brunswick, NJ: Rutgers Center of Alcohol Studies.

Hindmarch, I. (1980). Psychomotor function and psychoactive drugs. *British Journal of Clinical Pharmacology, 10,* 189–209.

Hoffman, B. (1977, June/July). The case against alcohol. *Strength and Health, 45,* 62–63.

Holder, H.D. (1987). Alcoholism treatment and potential health care cost saving. *Medical Care, 25*(1), 52–71.

Holder, H.D., & Blose, J.O. (1992). The reduction of health care costs associated with alcoholism treatment: A 14-year longitudinal study. *Journal of Studies on Alcohol, 53,* 293–302.

Horton, D. (1991). Alcohol use in primitive societies. In D.J. Pittman & H.R. White (Eds.), *Society, culture, and drinking patterns reexamined* (pp. 7–31). New Brunswick, NJ: Rutgers Center of Alcohol Studies.

Houmard, J.A., Langenfeld, M.E., Wiley, R.L., & Siefert, J. (1987). Effects of the acute ingestion of small amounts of alcohol on 5–mile run times. *Journal of Sports Medicine and Physical Fitness* (Torino, Italy), *27*, 253–257.

Hover, S., & Gaffney, L.R. (1991). The relationship between social skills and adolescent drinking. *Alcohol & Alcoholism, 26*, 207–214.

Howat, P., Sleet, D., & Smith, I. (1991). Alcohol and driving: Is the 0.05% blood alcohol concentration limit justified? *Drug and Alcohol Review, 10*, 151–166.

Hunt, W.A., Barnett, L.W., & Branch, L.G. (1971). Relapse rates in addiction programs. *Journal of Clinical Psychology, 27*, 455–456.

Impellizzeri, M.T. (1988, March/April). Who's the best sport? The designated driver. *Alcoholism and Addiction, 8*, 44–45.

Indian Health Service. (1991). *Trends in Indian health, 1991*. Rockville, MD: Author.

Institute of Medicine. (1990). *Broadening the base of treatment for alcohol problems*. Washington, DC: National Academy Press.

Jacobson, G.R. (1983). Detection, assessment, and diagnosis of alcoholism: Current techniques. In M. Galanter (Ed.), *Recent developments in alcoholism: Vol. 1. Genetics, behavioral treatment, social mediators and prevention, current concepts in diagnostics* (pp. 377–413). New York: Plenum Press.

Jellinek, E.M. (1977). The symbolism of drinking: A culture-historical approach. *Journal of Studies on Alcohol, 38*, 849–866.

Johnson, C.A., Pentz, M.A., Weber, M.D., Dwyer, J.H., Baer, N., Mackinnon, D.P., Hansen, W.B., & Flay, B.R. (1990). Relative effectiveness of comprehensive community programming for drug abuse prevention with high-risk and low-risk adolescents. *Journal of Consulting and Clinical Psychology, 58*, 447–456.

Johnson, E.M., Amatetti, S., Funkhouser, J.E., & Johnson, S. (1988). Theories and models supporting prevention approaches to alcohol problems among youth. *Public Health Reports, 103*, 578–586.

Johnson, R.C., Schwitters, S.Y., Wilson, J.R., Nagoshi, C.T., & McClearn, G.E. (1985). A cross-ethnic comparison of reasons given for using alcohol, not using alcohol, or ceasing to use alcohol. *Journal of Studies on Alcohol, 46*, 283–288.

Johnson, W.D. (1991). Predisposition to emotional distress and psychiatric illness amongst doctors: The role of unconscious and experiential factors. *British Journal of Medical Psychology, 64*, 317–329.

Johnson, W.O. (1988, August 8). Sports and suds: The beer business and the sports world have brewed up a potent partnership. *Sports Illustrated, 69*, 68–82.

Johnson, W.O. (1993, July 5). The agony of victory. *Sports Illustrated, 79*, 30–32, 34, 37.

Johnston, L.D., O'Malley, P.M., & Bachman, J.G. (1993). *National survey results on drug use from the monitoring the future project, 1975–1992:*

Volume 1: Secondary school students (NIH Publication No. 93–3597). Washington, DC: U.S. Government Printing Office.

Johnston, L.D., O'Malley, P.M., & Bachman, J.G. (1994). *National survey results on drug use from the monitoring the future study, 1975–1993: Volume I: Secondary school students,* (NIH Publication No. 94–3809). Washington, DC: U.S. Government Printing Office.

Johnston, L.D., O'Malley, P.M., & Bachman, J.G. (1995). *National survey results on drug use from the monitoring the future study, 1975–1994: Volume I: Secondary school students,* (NIH Publication No. 95-4026). Washington, DC: U.S. Government Printing Office.

Johnston, L.D., O'Malley, P.M., & Bachman, J.G. (1996). *National survey results on drug use from the monitoring the future study, 1975–1994: Volume II: College students and young adults* (NIH Publication No. 96–4027). Washington, DC: U.S. Government Printing Office.

Jokl, E. (1968). Notes on doping. In E. Jokl (Series Ed.) & E. Jokl & P. Jokl (Vol. Eds.), *Medicine and sport: Vol. 1. Exercise and altitude* (pp. 55–57). Basel, Switzerland: S. Karger.

Jonah, B.A. (1990). Psychosocial characteristics of impaired drivers: An integrated review in relation to problem behavior theory. In R.J. Wilson & R.E. Mann (Eds.), *Drinking and driving: Advances in research and prevention* (pp. 13–41). New York: Guilford Press.

Kandel, D.B. (1980). Drug and drinking behavior among youth. In A. Inkeles, N.J. Smelser, & R.H. Turner (Eds.), *Annual review of sociology: Vol. 6* (pp. 235–285). Palo Alto, CA: Annual Reviews.

Kandel, D.B., Yamaguchi, K., & Chen, K. (1992). Stages of progression in drug involvement from adolescence to adulthood: Further evidence for the gateway theory. *Journal of Studies on Alcohol, 53,* 447–457.

Karvinin, E., Miettinen, M., & Ahlman, K. (1962). Physical performance during hangover. *Quarterly Journal of Studies on Alcohol, 23,* 208–215.

Kazdin, A.E. (1993). Adolescent mental health: Prevention and treatment programs. *American Psychologist, 48,* 127–141.

Kimmel, W.A. (1993). *Need, demand, and problem assessment for substance abuse services* (Technical Assistance Publication Series No. 3). Rockville, MD: Substance Abuse and Mental Health Services Administration, Center for Substance Abuse Treatment.

Kivlahan, D.R., Marlatt, G.A., Fromme, K., Coppel, D.B., & Williams, E. (1990). Secondary prevention with college drinkers: Evaluation of an alcohol skills training program. *Journal of Consulting and Clinical Psychology, 58,* 805–810.

Klein, H. (1991). Cultural determinants of alcohol use in the United States. In D.J. Pittman & H.R. White (Eds.), *Society, culture, and drinking patterns reexamined* (pp. 114–134). New Brunswick, NJ: Rutgers Center of Alcohol Studies.

Koller, W.C., & Biary, N. (1984). Effects of alcohol on tremors. Comparison with propranolol. *Neurology, 34,* 221–222.

Kozlowski, J.C. (1989). Minnesota ski resort failure to supervise intoxicated skier. *Recreation and Parks Law Report, 6* (3), 100–101.

Kreitman, N. (1986). Alcohol consumption and the prevention paradox. *British Journal of Addiction, 81,* 353–363.

Krentzman, J. (1991, July). Baseball's top relief pitcher is grateful for a second chance at life. *Sober Times, 5,* 22–23.

Lemert, E.M. (1991). Alcohol, values, and social control. In D.J. Pittman & H.R. White (Eds.), *Society, culture, and drinking patterns reexamined* (pp. 681–701). New Brunswick NJ: Rutgers Center of Alcohol Studies.

Lesser known medical consequences of alcohol (1993) *Alcohol Health & Research World 17* (4).

Lester, D. (1988). Genetic theory—An assessment of the heritability of alcoholism. In C.D. Chaudron & D.A. Wilkinson (Eds.), *Theories on alcoholism* (pp. 1–28). Toronto: Addiction Research Foundation.

Lettieri, D.J. (1987). Stress and stages of addiction. In E. Gottheil, K.A. Druley, S. Pashko, & S.P. Weinstein (Eds.), *Stress and addiction* (pp. 270–282). New York: Brunner/Mazel.

Lewis, D.C., & Gordon, A.J. (1983). Alcoholism and the general hospital: The Roger Williams intervention program. *Bulletin of the New York Academy of Medicine, 59* (2), 181–197.

Lewis, D.C., Niven, R.G., Czechowicz, D., & Trumble, J.G. (1987). A review of medical education in alcohol and other drug abuse. *JAMA 257,* 2945–2948.

Lewis, J.F., James, R.J., Hastings, S.C., & Ford, J.J. (1992). *Drug and alcohol abuse in the schools: A practical guide for administrators and educators for combatting drug and alcohol abuse* (2nd ed.). Topeka, KS: National Organization on Legal Problems for Education.

Lewy, R. (1986). Alcoholism in house staff physicians: An occupational hazard. *Journal of Occupational Medicine, 28* (2), 79–81.

Lex, B.W. (1987). Review of alcohol problems in ethnic minority groups. *Journal of Consulting and Clinical Psychology, 55,* 293–300.

Leyshon, G.A. (1976, January). Alcohol and the athlete. Bulletin—*Coaching Association of Canada Bulletin, 5,* 19–20.

Lieber, J. (1993, January 11). Image of hope: John Lucas, the new coach of the San Antonio Spurs, sees himself as an example for recovering addicts. *Sports Illustrated, 78,* 46–48, 51.

Linnoila, M., & Mattila, M.J. (1973). Drug interaction on psychomotor skills related to driving: Diazepam and alcohol. *European Journal of Clinical Pharmacology, 5,* 186–194.

Litt, M.D., Babor, T.F., DelBoca, F.K., Kadden, R.M., & Cooney, N.L. (1992). Types of alcoholics, II: Application of an empirically derived typology to treatment matching. *Archives of General Psychiatry, 49,* 609–614.

Live and learn: Maybe this accident is a blessing in disguise (1991, May 20). *Sports Illustrated, 74,* 21.

Lockwood, A., & Saunders, B. (1993). What prevents prevention? Lessons from the failure of a university alcohol and drug policy. *Australian Journal of Public Health, 17* (2), 91–95.

Lorion, R.P., Bussell, D., & Goldberg, R. (1991). Identification of youth at high risk for alcohol or other drug problems. In E.N. Goplerud (Ed.), *Preventing adolescent drug use: From theory to practice* (pp. 53–89) (DHHS Publication No. ADM 91–1725). Rockville, MD: Office for Substance Abuse Prevention.

Lowcock, P., Cook, D.L., & Tricker, R. (1992, Fall). The drugs in sport education program at the University of Kansas. *Association for the Advancement of Applied Sport Psychology Newsletter, 7*, 10.

MacAndrew, C., & Edgerton, R.B. (1969). *Drunken comportment: A social explanation.* Chicago: Aldine.

Malone, D.L. (1991). The nature and extent of drug and alcohol use within a professional sports league (Doctoral dissertation, University of Pittsburgh, 1991). *Dissertation Abstracts International, 52*, 2823A.

Mangum, M., Gatch, W., Cocke, T.B., & Brooks, E. (1986). The effects of beer consumption on physiological responses to submaximal exercise. *Journal of Sports Medicine and Physical Fitness* (Torino, Italy), *26*, 301–305.

Mannaioni, P.F. (1984). *Clinical pharmacology of drug dependence.* Padua, Italy: Piccin.

Manno, B.R., & Manno, J.E. (1988). Epidemiologic basis of alcohol psychomotor performance impairment. In J.C. Garriott (Ed.), *Medicolegal aspects of alcohol determination in biological specimens* (pp. 245–271). Littleton, MA: PSG.

Mantle, M., & Lieber, J. (1994, April 18). Time in a bottle: After 42 years of alcohol abuse, a legendary ballplayer describes his life of self-destructive behavior and hopes his recovery will finally make him a true role model. *Sports Illustrated, 80*, 66–72, 74, 76–77.

Marlatt, G.A. (1987). Alcohol, the magic elixir: Stress, expectancy and the transformation of emotional states. In C.R. Figley (Series Ed.) & E. Gotth0eil, K.A. Druley, S. Pashko, & S.P. Weinstein (Vol. Eds.), *Brunner/Mazel psychosocial stress series: Vol. 9 Stress and addiction* (pp 302–322). New York: Brunner/Mazel.

Marlatt, G.A. (1988). Research on behavioral strategies for the prevention of alcohol problems. *Contemporary Drug Problems, 15*, 31–45.

Marlatt, G.A., Larimer, M.E., Baer, J.S., & Quigley, L.A. (1993). Harm reduction for alcohol problems: Moving beyond the controlled drinking controversy. *Behavior Therapy, 24*, 461–504.

Masia, S. (1978, November). So you're gonna ski the big ones: Be in shape, cool it the first day, eat well, and ease off at the bar. *Ski, 43*, 161.

Mason, D.T., Lusk, M.W., & Gintzler, M. (1992). Beyond ideology in drug policy: The primary prevention model. *The Journal of Drug Issues, 22*, 959–976.

Mathew, R.J., Wilson, W.H., Blazer, D.G., & George, L.K. (1993). Psychiatric disorders in adult children of alcoholics: Data from the Epidemiologic Catchment Area project. *American Journal of Psychiatry, 150*, 793–800.

May, P.A. (1989). Alcohol abuse and alcoholism among American Indians: An overview. In T.D. Watts & R. Wright (Eds.), *Alcoholism in minority populations* (pp. 95–119). Springfield, IL: Charles C. Thomas.

McAuliffe, W.E., Rohman, M., Breer, P., Wyshak, G., Santangelo, S., & Magnuson, E. (1991). Alcohol use and abuse in random samples of physicians and medical students. *American Journal of Public Health, 81,* 177–182.

McGinnis, J.M., & Foege, W.H. (1993). Actual causes of death in the United States. *JAMA, 270,* 2207–2212.

McKnight, A.J. (1993). Server intervention: Accomplishments and needs. *Alcohol Health & Research World, 17,* 76–83.

McLellan, A.T., Erdlen, F.R., Erdlen, D.L., & O'Brien, C.P. (1981). Psychological severity and response to alcoholism rehabilitation. *Drug and Alcohol Dependence, 8,* 23–35.

McNaughton, L., & Preece, D. (1986). Alcohol and its effects on sprint and middle distance running. *British Journal of Sports Medicine, 20* (2), 56–59.

Mikow, V.A., & Raven, M.R. (1993). *North Carolina student athletes' and non-athletes' use of and beliefs about alcohol and other drugs.* Raleigh, NC: North Carolina Department of Public Instruction, Alcohol and Drug Defense Section.

Miller, W.R. (1984). Teaching responsible drinking skills. In P.M. Miller & T.D. Nirenberg (Eds.), *Prevention of alcohol abuse* (pp. 371–385). New York: Plenum Press.

Miller, W.R. (1989a). Follow-up assessment. In R.K. Hester & W.R. Miller (Eds.), *Handbook of alcoholism treatment approaches: Effective alternatives* (pp. 81–89). New York: Pergamon Press.

Miller, W.R. (1989b). Matching individuals with interventions. In R.K. Hester & W.R. Miller (Eds.), *Handbook of alcoholism treatment approaches: Effective alternatives* (pp. 261–271). New York: Pergamon Press.

Miller, W.R. (1990). Alcohol treatment alternatives: What works? In H.B. Milkman & L.I. Sederer (Eds.), *Treatment choices for alcoholism and substance abuse* (pp. 253–264). New York: Lexington Books.

Miller, W.R., Benefield, R.G., & Tonigan, J.S. (1993). Enhancing motivation for change in problem drinking: A controlled comparison of two therapist styles. *Journal of Consulting and Clinical Psychology, 61,* 455–461.

Miller, W.R., & Hester, R.K. (1986a). The effectiveness of alcoholism treatment: What research reveals. In W.R. Miller & N. Heather (Eds.), *Treating addictive behaviors: Processes of change* (pp. 121–174). New York: Plenum Press.

Miller, W.R., & Hester, R.K. (1986b). Inpatient alcoholism treatment: Who benefits? *American Psychologist, 16,* 794–805.

Miller, W.R., & Hester, R.K. (1986c). Matching problem drinkers with optimal treatments. In W.R. Miller & N. Heather (Eds.), *Treating addictive behaviors: Processes of change* (pp. 175–204). New York: Plenum Press.

Miller, W.R., & Rollnick, S. (1991). *Motivational interviewing: Preparing people to change addictive behavior.* New York: Guilford Press.

Miller, W.R., & Sanchez, V.C. (1994). Motivating young adults for treatment and lifestyle change. In G.S. Howard & P.E. Nathan (Eds.), *Alcohol use and misuse by young adults.* South Bend, IN: University of Notre Dame.

Mirkin, G. (1981, June). Alcohol and running: A sober look at some of the scientific data. *The Runner, 3,* 14.

Mitchell, M. C. (1985). Alcohol-induced impairment of central nervous system function: Behavioral skills involved in driving. *Journal of Studies on Alcohol, Supplement 10,* 109–116.

Monarca, S., Donato, F., Modolo, M.A., Brunelli, L., Spiazzi, R., Pasquale, L., & Nardi, G. (1991). Drinking habits among high school students in Perugia, Italy, in 1981 and 1988: Time trends and correlates. *The International Journal of the Addictions, 26,* 1107–1122.

Monti, P.M., Gulliver, S.B., Myers, M.G. (1994). Social skills training for alcoholics: Assessment and treatment. *Alcohol & Alcoholism 29,* 627–637.

Moore, R.D., Bone, L.R., Geller, G., Mamon, J.A., Stokes, E.J., & Levine, D.M. (1989). Prevalence, detection, and treatment of alcoholism in hospitalized patients. *JAMA, 261,* 403–407.

Moore, R.D., Mead, L., & Pearson, T.A. (1990). Youthful precursors of alcohol abuse in physicians. *The American Journal of Medicine 88,* 332–336.

Moskowitz, H., & Burns, M. (1990). Effects of alcohol on driving performance. *Alcohol Health & Research World, 14,* 12–14.

Moskowitz, H., Burns, M.M., & Williams, A.F. (1985). Skills performance at low blood alcohol levels. *Journal of Studies on Alcohol, 46,* 482–485.

Nack, W. (1993, April 19). From fame to shame. *Sports Illustrated, 78,* 70–82.

National Institute on Alcohol Abuse and Alcoholism. (July, 1990). Children of alcoholics: Are they different? *Alcohol Alert* (No. 9, PH288). Rockville, MD: Author.

National Institute on Alcohol Abuse and Alcoholism. (July, 1993). Alcohol and cancer. *Alcohol Alert* (No. 21, PH345). Rockville, MD: Author.

Nattiv, A., & Puffer, J.C. (1991). Lifestyles and health risks of collegiate athletes. *The Journal of Family Practice, 33,* 585–590.

Nelson, J. (1991, May 16). Nothing beats a game for beer ads. *The Houston Post,* pp. B1, B12.

New Jersey: Consumption of alcohol at football games leads to litigation after injury occurs. (1987, Fall). *Sports and the Courts, 8,* 2–3.

Newcomb, M.D., & Bentler, P.M. (1988). *Consequences of adolescent drug use: Impact on the lives of young adults.* Newbury Park, CA: Sage.

Nightingale, D. (1981, November 21). Drugs, alcohol major headache in pro leagues. *The Sporting News, 192,* 13–14.

Nuotto, E., & Mattila, M.J. (1990). Actions and interactions of alcohol on performance tests. In S. Parvez & H. Parvez (Series Eds.) & H. Ollat, S. Parvez, & H. Parvez (Vol. Eds.), *Progress in alcohol research: Volume 2. Alcohol and behaviour: Basic and clinical aspects* (pp. 117–129). Utrecht, The Netherlands: VSP.

Nuzzo, N.A., & Waller, D.P. (1988). Drug abuse in athletes. In J.A. Thomas (Ed.), *Drugs, athletes, and physical performance* (pp. 141–167). New York: Plenum.

Oberman, J.P. (1989, October). Student athletes work toward a drug-free school. *Journal of the New York State School Boards Association,* 19–20.

O'Boyle, M. (1993). Personality disorder and multiple substance dependence. *Journal of Personality Disorders, 7,* 342–347.

O'Brien, C.P. (1993). Alcohol and sport: Impact of social drinking on recreational and competitive sports performance [Guest Editorial]. *Sports Medicine, 15,* 71–77.

Ogilvie, B.C. (1987). Counseling for sports career termination. In J.R. May & M.J. Asken (Eds.), *Sport psychology: The psychological health of the athlete* (pp. 213–230). New York: PMA.

Ohio-wrestling after drinking costs high school senior. (1991). *Sports and the Courts, 12* (1), 1–2.

Orcutt, J.D. (1991). The social integration of beers and peers: Situational contingencies in drinking and intoxication. In D.J. Pittman & H.R. White (Eds.), *Society, culture, and drinking patterns reexamined* (pp. 198–215). New Brunswick, NJ: Rutgers Center of Alcohol Studies.

Overman, S.J., & Terry, T. (1991). Alcohol use and attitudes: A comparison of college athletes and nonathletes. *Journal of Drug Education, 21* (2), 107–117.

Palmer, J., Davis, E., Sher, A., & Hicks, S. (1989). High school senior athletes as peer educators and role models: An innovative approach to drug prevention. *Journal of Alcohol and Drug Education, 35* (1), 23–27.

Parry-Jones, D. (1980, October). Is rugby on the path of soccer? *Rugby World, 20,* 51.

Parsons, O.A. (1986). Cognitive functioning in sober social drinkers: A review and critique. *Journal of Studies on Alcohol, 47,* 101–114.

Parsons, O.A., Butters, N., & Nathan, P.E. (Eds.) (1987). *Neuropsychology of alcoholism: Implications for diagnosis and treatment.* New York: Guilford Press.

Parsons, O.A., & Leber, W.R. (1981). The relationship between cognitive dysfunction and brain damage in alcoholics: Causal, interactive, or epiphenomenal? *Alcoholism: Clinical and Experimental Research, 5,* 326–343.

Partanen, J., & Montonen, M. (1988). *Alcohol and the mass media.* Copenhagen, Denmark: World Health Organization.

Pollard, A., Abraham, T., & Douglas, R.R. (1989, December). Avoiding litigation: Elliot Lake's alcohol management policy. *Recreation Canada, 47* (5), 12–18.

Porterfield, D. (1987, July/August). Alcohol and skiing: Drinking and driving don't mix. But how does alcohol affect water skiers? AWSA's safety committee found conclusive answers. *The Water Skier, 37,* 78–80.

Postman, N., Nystrom, C., Strate, L., & Weingartner, C. (1987). *Myths, men, & beer: An analysis of beer commercials on broadcast television, 1987.* Washington, DC: AAA Foundation for Traffic Safety.

Prentice, D.A., & Miller, D.T. (1993). Pluralistic ignorance and alcohol use on campus: Some consequences of misperceiving the social norm. *Journal of Personality and Social Psychology, 64,* 243–256.

Prevention of alcohol-related problems. (1993). *Alcohol Health & Research World, 17* (1).

Prochaska, J.O., DiClemente, C.C., & Norcross, J.C. (1992). In search of how people change: Applications to addictive behaviors. *American Psychologist, 47,* 1102–1114.

Puff, puff—guzzle, guzzle—how smoking and drinking affect your game. (1982, May). *National Racquetball, 11,* 36–38.

Pyorala, E. (1990). Trends in alcohol consumption in Spain, Portugal, France, and Italy from the 1950s until the 1980s. *British Journal of Addiction, 85,* 469–477.

Rassool, G.H. (1993). Nursing and substance misuse: Responding to the challenge. *Journal of Advanced Nursing, 18,* 1401–1407.

Ray, O., & Ksir, C. (1993). *Drugs, society, & human behavior.* St. Louis: Mosby.

Regier, D.A., Narrow, W.E., Rae, D.S., Manderscheid, R.W., Locke, B.Z., & Goodwin, F.K. (1993). The de facto U.S. mental and addictive disorders service system: Epidemiologic catchment area prospective 1-year prevalence rates of disorders and services. *Archives of General Psychiatry, 50,* 85–94.

Reichman, W., Young, D.W., & Gracin, L. (1988). Identification of alcoholics in the workplace. In M. Galanter (Ed.), *Recent development in alcoholism: Vol. 6* (pp. 171–179). New York: Plenum Press.

Reilly, R. (1987, November 23). In search of trust: Dexter Manley of the Redskins thought the world had betrayed him—until he faced his daughter's illness and his own alcoholism. *Sports Illustrated, 67,* 84–88, 90–94.

Reilly, R. (1993, June 7). Sweet redemption: John Daly, now chugging M & M's instead of beers, is confining his hard-driving ways to the golf course. *Sports Illustrated, 78,* 66–72, 74–76, 79.

Reilly, T., & Halliday, F. (1985). Influence of alcohol ingestion on tasks related to archery. *Journal of Human Ergology, 14* (2), 99–104.

Research & Forecasts (1983). *The Miller Lite report on American attitudes toward sport.* Milwaukee: Miller Brewing.

Rhoades, E.R., Mason, R.D., Eddy, P., Smith, E.M., & Burns, T.R. (1988). The Indian Health Service approach to alcoholism among American Indians and Alaska Natives. *Public Health Reports, 103,* 621–627.

Rice, D.P. (1993). The economic cost of alcohol abuse and alcohol dependence: 1990. *Alcohol Health & Research World, 17,* 10–11.

Ringwalt, C. (1988). *Student athletes and non-athletes: Do their use of and beliefs about alcohol and other drugs differ? A special research report.* Raleigh, NC: North Carolina Department of Public Instruction, Alcohol and Drug Defense Division.

Roche, A.M., & Richard, G.P. (1991). Doctors' willingness to intervene in patients' drug and alcohol problems. *Social Science and Medicine, 33,* 1053–1061.

Roman, P.M. (1988a). Biological features of women's alcohol use: A review. *Public Health Reports, 103,* 628–637.

Roman, P.M. (1988b). Growth and transformation in workplace alcoholism programming: In M. Galanter (Ed.), *Recent developments in alcoholism: Volume 6* (pp. 131–158). New York: Plenum.

Romney, D.M., & Bynner (1985). Hospital staff's perceptions of the alcoholic. *The International Journal of the Addictions, 20,* 393–402.

Rooney, J.F. (1984). Sports and clean living: A useful myth? *Drug and Alcohol Dependence, 13* (1), 75–87.

Ross, H.E., Glaser, F.B., & Germanson, T. (1988). The prevalence of psychiatric disorders in patients with alcohol and other drug problems. *Archives of General Psychiatry, 45,* 1023 1031.

Ryan, B.E., & Mosher, J.F. (1991). *Progress report: Alcohol promotion on campus.* San Rafael, CA: Marin Institute for the Prevention of Alcohol and Other Drug Problems.

Salo, D.C. (1988, August). A physiological look at alcohol. *Swimming World and Junior Swimming, 29,* 21–22.

Saxe, L., Dougherty, D., Esty, K., & Fine, M. (1983). *The effectiveness and costs of alcoholism treatment.* Washington, DC: U.S. Congress, Office of Technology Assessment.

Schiavi, R.C. (1990). Chronic alcoholism and male sexual dysfunction. *Journal of Sex and Marital Therapy, 16,* 23–33.

Sharp, D.J., & Lowe, G. (1989). Adolescents and alcohol—A review of the recent British research. *Journal of Adolescence, 12,* 295–307.

Shephard, R.J. (1972). *Alive man: The physiology of physical activity.* Springfield, IL: Charles C Thomas.

Siegel, B.J., & Fitzgerald, F.T. (1988). A survey on the prevalence of alcoholism among the faculty and house staff of an academic teaching hospital. *The Western Journal of Medicine, 148,* 593–595.

Single, E. W. (1987). The control of public drinking: The impact of the environment on alcohol problems. In N.K. Mello (Series Ed.) & H.D. Holder (Vol. Ed.), *Advances in substance abuse: Behavioral and biological research: Supplement 1. Control issues in alcohol abuse prevention: Strategies for states and communities* (pp. 219–232). Greenwich, CT: JAI Press.

Single, E.W. (1988). The availability theory of alcohol-related problems. In C.D. Chaudron & D.A. Wilkinson (Eds.), *Theories on alcoholism* (pp. 325–351). Toronto: Addiction Research Foundation.

Skinner, H.A. (1984). Assessing alcohol use by patients in treatment. In R.G. Smart, H.D. Cappell, F.B. Glaser, Y. Israel, H. Kalant, R.E. Popham, W. Schmidt, & E.M. Sellers (Eds.), *Research advances in alcohol and drug problems: Vol. 8* (pp. 183–207). New York: Plenum.

Skinner, H.A. (1986). Early intervention for alcohol and drug problems: Core issues for medical education. *Australian Drug and Alcohol Review, 5,* 69–74.

Smart, R. (1988). Does alcohol advertising affect overall consumption? A review of empirical studies. *Journal of Studies on Alcohol, 49,* 314–323.

Smith, D.L. (1979, February). Caffeine, alcohol, and aspirin. Don't put a beer bottle in your water bottle carrier, even if it fits. *Bicycling, 20,* 18.

Smith, G. (1993, July 12). The ripples from little Lake Nellie: Four months after Cleveland Indians pitchers Tim Crews and Steve Olin died in a boating accident, their families and friends are coming to grips with the grief that still washes over them. *Sports Illustrated, 79,* 18–28, 31.

Sobell, L.C., & Sobell, M.B. (1990). Self-report issues in alcohol abuse: State of the art and future directions. *Behavioral Assessment, 12* (1), 77–90.

Sobell, L.C., Sobell, M.B., Riley, D.M., Klajner, F., Leo, G.I., Pavan, D., & Cancilla, A. (1986). Effect of television programming and advertising on alcohol consumption in normal drinkers. *Journal of Studies on Alcohol, 47,* 333–340.

Sobell, L.C., Sobell, M.B., Toneatto, T., & Leo, G.I. (1993). What triggers the resolution of alcohol problems without treatment? *Alcoholism: Clinical and Experimental Research, 17,* 217–224.

Spicer, J. (1993). *The Minnesota model: The evolution of the multidisciplinary approach to addiction recovery.* Center City, MN: Hazelden Foundation.

Stainback, R.D., & Rogers, R.W. (1983). Identifying effective components of alcohol abuse prevention programs: Effects of fear appeals, message style, and source expertise. *The International Journal of the Addictions, 18,* 393–405.

Stall, R. (1986). Change and stability in quantity and frequency of alcohol use among aging males: A 19-year follow-up study. *British Journal of Addiction, 81,* 537–544.

Stewart, L. (1981, March). The drink of choice among runners: Beer. *Runner's World, 16,* 68–71.

Stuck, M.F. (1988). Belief and behavior: Sport and clean living. *Arena Review, 12* (1), 13–24.

Stuck, M.F. (1990). *Adolescent worlds: Drug use and athletic activity.* New York: Praeger.

Substance Abuse and Mental Health Services Administration. (1992). *CSAP national evaluation of the community partnership demonstration program: Second annual report: Executive summary* (Contract No. 277-90-2003). Rockville, MD: Author, Center for Substance Abuse Prevention.

Substance Abuse and Mental Health Services Administration. (1995). *National household survey on drug abuse: Main findings 1993* (DHHS Publication No. SMA 95-3020). Rockville, MD: Author.

Sue, D. (1987). Use and abuse of alcohol by Asian Americans. *Journal of Psychoactive Drugs, 19*, 57–66.

Sullivan, E.J., & Handley, S.M. (1992). Alcohol and drug abuse in nurses. *Annual Review of Nursing Research, 10*, 113–125.

Sutherland, V.J., & Cooper, C.L. (1993). Identifying distress among general practitioners: Predictors of psychological ill-health and job dissatisfaction. *Social Science and Medicine, 37*, 575–581.

Svendsen, R., Griffin, T., & McIntyre, D.E. (Eds.) (1984). *Chemical health: School athletics and fine arts activities.* Center City, MN: Hazelden Foundation.

Sweeney, M.R. (1988). The propensity for alcohol misuse among collegiate football players: Its relationship to athletic success, psychological profile, and family of origin (Doctoral dissertation, University of Missouri-Kansas City, 1987). *Dissertation Abstracts International, 48*, 2838A.

Tabakoff, B., & Hoffman, P.L. (1988). A neurobiological theory of alcoholism. In C.D. Chaudron & D.A. Wilkinson (Eds.), *Theories on alcoholism* (pp. 29–72). Toronto: Addiction Research Foundation.

Tabakoff, B., & Petersen, R.C. (1988). Brain damage and alcoholism. *The Counselor, 6*(5), 13–16.

Tanny, A. (1986, June). Booze: How it works on your liver, your muscles, your heart. *Muscle and Fitness, 47*, 47, 158–159.

Tarter, R.E. (1985). Neurobehavioral correlates of alcoholism vulnerability. In N.C. Chang & H.M. Chao (Eds.), *Early identification of alcohol abuse: Proceedings of a workshop* (Research Monograph No. 17., pp. 149–167) Rockville, MD: National Institute on Alcohol Abuse and Alcoholism.

Tarter, R.E., Alterman, A.I., & Edwards, K.L. (1988). Neurobehavioral theory of alcoholism etiology. In C.D. Chaudron & D.A. Wilkinson (Eds.), *Theories on alcoholism* (pp. 73–102). Toronto: Addiction Research Foundation.

Tarter, R.E. & Edwards, K.L. (1986). Antecedents to alcoholism: Implications for prevention and treatment. *Behavior Therapy, 17*, 346–361.

Temple, M.T., & Fillmore, K.M. (1985–1986). The variability of drinking patterns and problems among young men, age 16–31: A longitudinal study. *The International Journal of the Addictions, 20*, 1595–1620.

Thomson, R.W. (1977). *Sport and deviance: A subcultural analysis.* Unpublished doctoral dissertation, University of Alberta, Edmonton.

Tipliski, V.M. (1993). The characteristics of recovering chemically-dependent Manitoba nurses. *The International Journal of the Addictions, 28*, 711–717.

Tricker, R., & Cook, D. (Eds.) (1993). *Athletes at risk: Drugs and sport.* Dubuque, IA: Brown & Benchmark.

Tricker, R., Cook, D.L., & McGuire, R. (1989). Issues related to drug abuse in college athletics: Athletes at risk. *The Sport Psychologist, 3,* 155–165.

Trinkoff, A.M., Eaton, W.W., & Anthony, J.C. (1991). The prevalence of substance abuse among registered nurses. *Nursing Research, 40,* 172–175.

Tuchfeld, B.S. (1981). Spontaneous remission in alcoholics: Empirical observations and theoretical implications. *Journal of Studies on Alcohol, 42,* 626–641.

Turrisi, R., Jaccard, J., Kelly, S.Q., & O'Malley, C.M. (1993). Social psychological factors involved in adolescents' efforts to prevent their friends from driving while intoxicated. *Journal of Youth and Adolescence, 22,* 147–169.

23 U.S.C.A.§158 (West 1990 & Supp. 1996).

U.S. Department of Commerce. (1992). *Statistical abstracts of the United States* (112th ed.). Washington, DC: U.S. Government Printing Office.

U.S. Department of Health and Human Services. (1990). *Seventh special report to the U.S. Congress on alcohol and health* (Contract No. ADM-281-88-0002). Rockville, MD: National Institute on Alcohol Abuse and Alcoholism.

U.S. Department of Health and Human Services. (1991). *Healthy people 2000: National health promotion and disease prevention objectives* (DHHS Publication No. PHS 91-50213). Washington, DC: U.S. Government Printing Office.

U.S. Department of Health and Human Services. (1993). *Eighth special report to the U.S. Congress on alcohol and health* (Contract No. ADM-281-91-0003). Rockville, MD: National Institute on Alcohol Abuse and Alcoholism.

U.S. General Accounting Office. (1992). *Adolescent drug use prevention: Common features of promising community programs* (GAO/PEMD-92-2). Washington DC: Author.

Umbricht-Schneiter, A., Santora, P., & Moore, R.D. (1991). Alcohol abuse: Comparison of two methods for assessing its prevalence and associated morbidity in hospitalized patients. *The American Journal of Medicine, 91,* 110–118.

Vaillant, G.E. (1983). *The natural history of alcoholism: Causes, patterns, and paths to recovery.* Cambridge, MA: Harvard University Press.

Valenti, J., & Naclerio, R. (1990). *Swee'Pea and other playground legends: Tales of drugs, violence, and basketball.* New York: Michael Kesend.

Vital Statistics. (1993, March). *The Edell Health Letter, 12,* 5.

Wadler, G.I. & Hainline, B. (1989). *Drugs and the athlete.* Philadelphia: F.A. Davis.

Wallack, L. (1983). Alcohol advertising reassessed: The public health perspective. In M. Grant, M. Plant, & A. Williams (Eds.), *Economics and alcohol: Consumption and controls* (pp. 243–248). New York: Gardner Press.

Ward, C. (1990, June). Fighting talk. *New Statesman & Society, 3,* 24–25.

Welch, B., & Vecsey, G. (1982). *Five o'clock comes early: A young man's battle with alcoholism.* New York: Morrow.

Werner, E.E. (1986). Resilient offspring of alcoholics: A longitudinal study from birth to age 18. *Journal of Studies on Alcohol, 47,* 34–40.

Wetzig, D.L. (1990). Sex-role conflict in female athletes: A possible marker for alcoholism. *Journal of Alcohol and Drug Education, 35* (3), 45–53.

White, H.R., Bates, M.E., & Johnson, V. (1991). Learning to drink: Familial, peer, and media influences. In D.J. Pittman & H.R. White (Eds.), *Society, culture, and drinking patterns reexamined* (pp. 177–197). New Brunswick, NJ: Rutgers Center of Alcohol Studies.

Williams, G.D., & DeBakey, S.F. (1992). Changes in levels of alcohol consumption: United States, 1983 to 1988. *British Journal of Addiction, 87,* 643–648.

Williams, G.D., Stinson, F.S., Stewart, S.L., and Dufour, M.C. (1995). *Apparent per capita alcohol consumption: National, state, and regional trends, 1977–1993* (NIAAA Surveillance Report No. 35). Bethesda, MD: National Institute on Alcohol Abuse and Alcoholism.

Williams, M.H. (1991). Alcohol, marijuana, and beta blockers. In D.R. Lamb & M.H. Williams (Eds.), *Perspectives in exercise science and sports medicine: Volume 4: Ergogenics—enhancement of performance in exercise and sport* (pp. 331–372). Dubuque, IA: Brown & Benchmark.

Williams, M.H. (1994). Physical activity, fitness, and substance misuse and abuse. In C. Bouchard, R.J. Shephard, & T. Stephens (Eds.), *Physical activity, fitness, and health* (pp. 898–915). Champaign, IL: Human Kinetics.

Wilmes, D. (1993, March/April). Prevention in the '90s: More than just good intentions. *Prevention Pipeline, 6,* 79–80.

Wilsnack, S.C. (1991). Sexuality and women's drinking: Findings from a U.S. national study. *Alcohol Health & Research World, 15,* 147–150.

Wilsnack, S.C., Klassen, A.D., Schur, B.E., & Wilsnack, R.W. (1991). Predicting onset and chronicity of women's problem drinking: A five-year longitudinal analysis. *American Journal of Public Health, 81,* 305 318.

Wilsnack, S.C., & Wilsnack, R.W. (1991). Epidemiology of women's drinking. *Journal of Substance Abuse, 3,* 133–157.

Wong, G.M. (1988, November). NCAA wins two: Alcohol liability limited. *Athletic Business, 12,* 18.

Wong, G.M., & Ensor, R.J. (1985, May). Torts and tailgates. *Athletic Business, 9,* 46–49.

Woolf, N.B. (1986). Recruit coaches and athletes to help battle drugs. *The American School Board Journal, 173* (2), 36.

World Health Organization. (1992). *The ICD-10 classification of mental and behavioral disorders: Clinical descriptions and diagnostic guidelines.* Geneva: Author.

Wynd, T. (1988, October/December). Alcohol: Its effect on athletes. *Sports Coach, 12,* 29–31.

Yesavage, J.A., & Leirer, V.O. (1986). Hangover effects on aircraft pilots 14 hours after alcohol ingestion: A preliminary report. *American Journal of Psychiatry, 143,* 1546–1550.

Young, D.S., & Young, D.B. (1989). Drug testing and student-athlete assistance programs in National Collegiate Athletic Association women's sports. *Journal of Applied Research in Coaching and Athletics, 4*(2), 94–108.

Zador, P.L. (1991). Alcohol-related relative risk of fatal driver injuries in relation to driver age and sex. *Journal of Studies on Alcohol, 52,* 302–310.

INDEX

A

Abstinence rates, 177-178
Accidents, 74
Acculturation, of Hispanics, 8-9
Acute gastritis, 52
Acute intervention, 150, 157
Administrators, prevention role of, 119-120
Adolescents. *See also* High-school athletes
  alcohol use rationale, 41-42
  and consumption patterns, 3, 6-7, 31-36, 178-179
  prevention training for, 118
  risk factors for, 22, 108
  screening of, 108
Advertising
  influence of, 114-115
  in sports, 27-31
Aerobic performance, alcohol effect on, 68
African Americans, and consumption patterns, 8
Aftercare, 149,150-151
Age, and alcohol use, 35, 178-179. *See also* Adolescents; Elderly
Aggression, 57
Aggressive behavior, alcohol effects on, 57
AIDS. *See* Human immunodeficiency virus (HIV) infection
Alcohol
  acute behavioral and cognitive effects of, 55-57
  and cancer, 53
  concentration of, 3
  diuretic effects of, 67
  effect on cardiovascular system, 49-51
  effect on central nervous system, 50-51, 54
  effect on fitness tests, 66-67
  effect on gastrointestinal system, 52
  effect on human performance, 58-62
  effect on immune system, 52-53
  effect on metabolism, 65-66
  effect on reproductive system, 52
  effect on sport performance, 63-66, 168
  effect on women, 54
  ergogenic effects, 63
  and fetal malformation, 53
  metabolism of, 48-49
  psychomotor effects, 58-62, 64-65
  tolerance of, 50

Alcohol abuse
  definition of, 2
  diagnosis of, 11-13, 93-96
  economic costs of, 10
  by high-profile athletes, 73-74
  incidence among athletes, 72-74
  incidence among sport professionals, 77-78
  and psychiatric disorders, 14-16
Alcohol dependence
  behavioral factors for, 22-23
  cognitive and behavioral effects of, 57-58
  composite description of, 6, 23
  definition of, 2
  diagnosis of, 11-13, 93-96
  etiology of, 16-21
  family history of, 21-22
  by high-profile athletes, 73-74
  incidence of, 4
  incidence among athletes, 72-74
  incidence among sport professionals, 77-78
  longitudinal studies of, 5-6
  men vs. women, 14-15
  natural history of, 128-129
  physical, 50-51
  predictors of, 6
  prevalence of, 14-15, 117
  and psychiatric disorders, 14-16
  psychological, 50
  risk factors for, 21-23, 166
Alcohol-flush reaction, definition of, 9
Alcohol use
  by adolescents, 3, 6-7, 31-36, 41-42, 178-179
  by athletes, 35-41
  attitude towards, 40-42
  by coaches, 43
  and consumption patterns, 3,4-5,6-7, 166, 176-177
  definition of, 2-3
  economic costs of, 10
  by the elderly, 7
  by ethnic groups, 7-10
  in Europe, 180-181
  guidelines for sports, 63-64, 69-70, 168
  by health professionals, 43
  history of, 3, 175-177
  incidence of, 4
  initiation of, 3-4
  military role of, 26
  parental influence on, 3-4
  peer group influence on, 3-4

ABOUT THE AUTHOR

Clinical and sport psychologist Robert D. Stainback, PhD, has more than 20 years of practical experience and research in substance abuse treatment. He has headed the Substance Abuse Treatment Program at the Birmingham Department of Veterans Affairs Medical Center in Birmingham, Alabama, and served as an assistant professor in psychology and psychiatry at the University of Alabama at Birmingham. His years of research and practical experience in the substance abuse treatment field include 12 years of directing treatment programs.

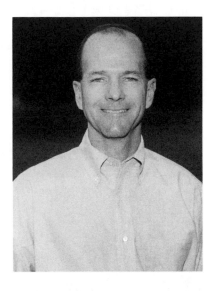

Stainback's shift in focus from addictions to health and sport psychology resulted from his experience as a Visiting Professor at the U.S. Olympic Training Center in 1988. He continued in this direction by serving as the sport psychologist for a U.S. Olympic athlete competing in the 1992 Winter Games.

The author lives in Birmingham with his wife, Judith La Marche. He enjoys reading and participating in aerobics and art classes.

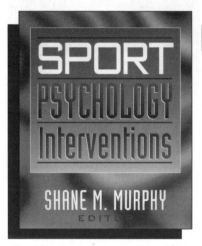
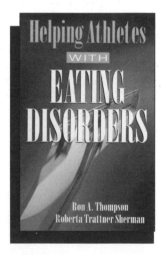